"This exceptionally rich book explores the multifaceted role and significance of the father in Lacan's work. Diego Londoño seamlessly connects logical formulations with socio-cultural reflections and clinical considerations, making this book not only a comprehensive discussion of Lacan's work but also a reference on how to apply it in contemporary practice."

Stijn Vanheule, *Ghent University*

"In *A Social Ontology of Psychosis*, Londoño provides a logical and genealogical account of the function and place of the father in civilization through a careful analysis of the various versions of the father in psychoanalytic theory as developed by Sigmund Freud and Jacques Lacan. His logico-genealogical reading of Lacan's theory of the Name-of-the-Father provides a contemporary commentary on psychotic subjectivity in civilization in both pathological and non-pathological forms. Moreover, in developing Lacan's theory of the Name-of-the-Father in relation to logic, set theory, the big Other, language and myth he provides an intriguing response to what may have occurred in Lacan's 1963 abandoned seminar, The Names of the Father."

Jonathan Redmond, *author*, Ordinary Psychosis and the Body

A Social Ontology of Psychosis

In *A Social Ontology of Psychosis*, Diego Enrique Londoño-Paredes explores how to interpret and apply the concept of the signifier of the Name-of-the-Father in Lacanian theory, particularly in the context of working with psychosis.

Londoño proposes a logical framework that draws on the work of Badiou, then traces the historical development of this concept and its implications as a structural necessity for anyone who speaks and engages in discourse. The book opens by exploring set theory, transitioning from nought to one, from the Thing to the object, essential for any presentation. Subsequently, it follows a historical path, examining the evolution of the figure and the signifier of the Father, journeying from ancient Mesopotamian roots through Modernity, and touching upon Claudel's theater and the films of the Coen brothers. Finally, it aligns Searle's social ontology with Lacan's discourses, highlighting psychosis as an illustration of being outside discourse, particularly when the Name-of-the-Father is foreclosed. Case material illustrates various ways that psychosis manifests without distinct clinical evidence.

This comprehensive book will be of great interest to practitioners and scholars in psychoanalysis, philosophy, the humanities, and the history of mental health and knowledge.

Diego Enrique Londoño-Paredes is a psychoanalyst and clinical psychologist from the Université Rennes 2, France, where he received his doctorate in psychology. He has been a professor in several psychology departments and is currently a member of the psychoanalytic association Analítica as well as Professor at the Universidad Nacional de Colombia and Universidad Manuela Beltrán.

The Lines of the Symbolic in Psychoanalysis Series

Series Editor:
Ian Parker, *Manchester Psychoanalytic Matrix*

Psychoanalytic clinical and theoretical work is always embedded in specific linguistic and cultural contexts and carries their traces, traces which this series attends to in its focus on multiple contradictory and antagonistic 'lines of the Symbolic'. This series takes its cue from Lacan's psychoanalytic work on three registers of human experience, the Symbolic, the Imaginary and the Real, and employs this distinctive understanding of cultural, communication and embodiment to link with other traditions of cultural, clinical and theoretical practice beyond the Lacanian symbolic universe. The Lines of the Symbolic in Psychoanalysis Series provides a reflexive reworking of theoretical and practical issues, translating psychoanalytic writing from different contexts, grounding that work in the specific histories and politics that provide the conditions of possibility for its descriptions and interventions to function. The series makes connections between different cultural and disciplinary sites in which psychoanalysis operates, questioning the idea that there could be one single correct reading and application of Lacan. Its authors trace their own path, their own line through the Symbolic, situating psychoanalysis in relation to debates which intersect with Lacanian work, explicating it, extending it and challenging it.

Philosophy After Lacan
Politics, Science, and Art
Edited by Alireza Taheri, Chris Vanderwees, and Reza Naderi

Critical Essays on the Drive
Lacanian Theory and Practice
Edited by Dan Collins and Eve Watson

A Social Ontology of Psychosis
Genea-logical Treatise on Lacan's Conception of Psychosis
Diego Enrique Londoño-Paredes

For more information about the series, please visit: https://www.routledge.com/The-Lines-of-the-Symbolic-in-Psychoanalysis-Series/book-series/KARNLOS

A Social Ontology of Psychosis

Genea-logical Treatise on Lacan's Conception of Psychosis

Diego Enrique Londoño-Paredes

Routledge
Taylor & Francis Group
LONDON AND NEW YORK

Designed cover image: © Getty Images

First published 2025
by Routledge
4 Park Square, Milton Park, Abingdon, Oxon OX14 4RN

and by Routledge
605 Third Avenue, New York, NY 10158

Routledge is an imprint of the Taylor & Francis Group, an informa business

British Library Cataloguing-in-Publication Data
A catalogue record for this book is available from the British Library

Library of Congress Cataloging-in-Publication Data
Names: Londoño-Paredes, Diego Enrique, author.
Title: A social ontology of psychosis : genea-logical treatise on Lacan's conception of psychosis / Diego Enrique Londoño-Paredes.
Description: Abingdon, Oxon ; New York, NY : Routledge, 2025. |
Series: The lines of the symbolic in psychoanalysis series |
Includes bibliographical references and index.
Identifiers: LCCN 2024025516 (print) |
LCCN 2024025517 (ebook) | ISBN 9781032663579 (hardback) |
ISBN 9781032663531 (paperback) | ISBN 9781032663616 (ebook)
Subjects: LCSH: Psychosis. | Lacan, Jacques, 1901–1981—Influence.
Classification: LCC RC512 .L54 2025 (print) |
LCC RC512 (ebook) | DDC 616.89—dc23/eng/20240614
LC record available at https://lccn.loc.gov/2024025516
LC ebook record available at https://lccn.loc.gov/2024025517

ISBN: 978-1-032-66357-9 (hbk)
ISBN: 978-1-032-66353-1 (pbk)
ISBN: 978-1-032-66361-6 (ebk)

DOI: 10.4324/9781032663616

Typeset in Times New Roman
by codeMantra

Contents

Series preface

This close reading, explication, extension, and contextualization of "psychosis" in Lacan's work provides the reader with a host of "points de capiton" for making sense of difficult texts. The reading is scholarly and faithful, working away at the interior space of what critics of Lacan suspect to be a hermetic closed field of psychoanalytic inquiry; indeed as hermetic and closed as the world of a subject diagnosed as "psychotic". This careful tracing of lines of argument, however, is precisely a way of tracing "lines of the symbolic", showing us the way psychoanalytic concepts are drawn from and then feed back into the symbolic universe we must inhabit and navigate in order to not be so diagnosed. Here is a case illustration of why the symbolic must be conceptualized as comprising many intersecting lines of attack, vantage points, and standpoints, instead of being comprised of a single worldview.

These lines are drawn out, explicated, and, from Lacan's work to later Lacanian psychoanalysts, they are displayed and explained. It is not easy to speak of such phenomena, which is why even many psychoanalysts resort to deceptively easy illustrations, conjuring up apparently easy-to-understand images in place of an attention to the array of signifiers that compose a concept. Diego Londoño avoids such a temptation to escape into the imaginary, and his explication is, instead, in and of the symbolic, of the language in which "psychotics" are spoken of.

A most difficult task in psychoanalysis, and not only psychoanalysis, is to contextualize what is so-often assumed to be one single worldview that is then, as a consequence, infused with imaginary content that would, it is hoped, fuse many contradictory lines of argument together. This impressive book takes on that task in order to provide, in place of forms of "psychogenesis"—developmental accounts of disorder so-beloved of so many psy professionals—a "social ontology of psychosis". Contextualization in psychoanalysis, whether focused on work with an analysand or as an analysis of the culture that gives rise to our theory and practice, must be historical, and this is why Lacan's conception of psychosis is here extended, written in the form of a genealogical treatise.

Just as there are many "Names-of-the-Father", many names that open out and question the patriarchal origins of psychoanalysis, so there are, we might say, many names of the real. One of those names is "history" itself, that which can be charted but never finally completely mapped, the territory for which there can, despite our attempts to imaginarize or symbolize it, be no full map.

Psychoanalytic clinical and theoretical work circulates through multiple intersecting antagonistic symbolic universes. This series opens connections between different cultural sites in which Lacanian work has developed in distinctive ways, in forms of work that question the idea that there could be single correct reading and application. The Lines of the Symbolic in Psychoanalysis series provides a reflexive reworking of psychoanalysis that transmits Lacanian writing from around the world, steering a course between the temptations of a metalanguage and imaginary reduction, between the claim to provide a god's eye view of psychoanalysis and the idea that psychoanalysis must everywhere be the same. The elaboration of psychoanalysis in the symbolic here grounds its theory and practice in the history and politics of the work in a variety of interventions that touch the real.

Ian Parker
Manchester Psychoanalytic Matrix

Introduction

Lacan published *Les complexes familiaux dans la formation de l'individu*, a text known as *La famille*, in 1938 at the request of Henri Wallon for the *Encyclopédie française*. In this text, he uses the concept of the *imago* to refer to a type of representation that mediates the infant's apprehension of reality and the objects of the world. Similarly, he uses the concept of the complex to refer to a time when these developing imagos become fixated, enabled by the image of a parental figure. The complex establishes everything from biological functions to emotions to adapted behavior with the object; it corresponds to the subject's rooting in the sociolinguistic world and its capture of reality. In terms of content, the complex represents an object; in terms of form, it is linked to a stage of objectification; and in terms of manifestation, it is an objective and affective form of knowledge and organization, as well as a reality-testing shock guided by a type of *loss* (Lacan, 1938).

Lacan declares the existence of three complexes: weaning, intrusion, and Oedipus. Each of these complexes favors a way of knowing the world and the objects the subject encounters, even if devoid of sufficient verbal baggage to name them. The baby disposes of images and bodily sensations, so physiological needs can be satisfied both by sight and by the sensation caused by the maternal breast and its nectar. The weaning complex comes into play when a first loss of the maternal object occurs, and the oral drive starts to operate as a relay for the presence/absence of that object. The second form of loss would be characterized by the arrival of a sibling or another child (cousin, nephew, etc.) into the family, thus giving place to the intrusion complex. This birth breaks with the privileged place and the attention that it enjoyed before the arrival of the newborn. A form of infantile jealousy is then established, which, despite what one may think, is very important for the development of sociability and knowledge. This new intruder does not only come to forge a sibling rivalry, but to underlie an imaginary identification. That is to say, the new brother or sister comes as an identifying other, as a double, an imago, "another as an object".

DOI: 10.4324/9781032663616-1

At the end of this section on the intrusion complex, Lacan links to it a very cherished subject of his: psychotic paranoia and the regressive logical time in delusional themes of a persecutory nature. The image of the intruder, the plunderer, the influencer is a form of regression or "connection" with the intrusion complex in paranoia.

> These connections are explained by the fact that the family group, reduced to the mother and siblings, outlines a psychic complex where reality tends to remain imaginary or, at most, abstract. The clinic shows that the impoverished group is certainly very favorable to the appearance of psychosis and that there we find most of the cases of shared delusions [*délires à deux*].
>
> (Lacan, 1938, p. 45 [*Translated by the author*])

For Lacan, the Mirror stage, *i.e.*, when the image of the body is formed and constituted as a unity, would favor understanding the relationship that the psychotic posits with the objects of the world. What remains of the Mirror stage and of the formation of the ego appears for the psychotic as "the fecund phase of delusion: a phase where objects, transformed by an ineffable strangeness, reveal themselves as shocks, enigmas, meanings. It is in this reproduction that the conformism, superficially assumed, by which the subject masked until then the narcissism of its relationship with reality collapses" (Lacan, 1938, p. 63). There would be an object that is not integrated as the satisfaction of desire; this object does not only represent an imago where the ego is constituted but also the ego-ideal, a third position in which Lacan recognizes the paternal imago. The object in psychosis would be deprived of the paternal imago, of its ideal. Lacan assumed this during his training days as a psychiatrist after attending many cases of shared delusions (*délires à deux*) that burst from "paranoid nests" or "pathogenic homes" (Claude, Migault, and Lacan, 1931; Lacan, 1931). For this reason, family complexes would come into play as reactions of the subject or as themes for delusions. Precisely, these themes are part of its structuring; they are intrinsic to the delusion itself and reveal not only its content but also its form.

Already, years before in his doctoral thesis, *De la psychose paranoïaque dans ses rapports avec la personnalité* (Lacan, 1932), Lacan explained how, in the delusions of interpretation, a "personal meaning" (morbid self-reference—Neisser's *krankhafte Eigenbeziehung*) of all events experienced by the psychotic predominates. A delusion of interpretation does not arise in a totally fortuitous way, as a simple arbitrariness of meaning, from random perceptions or from objects without affective significance, but is precisely composed of "relations of a social nature" that concern the psychotic itself. "The delusion of interpretation... is a delusion of the neighborhood, the street, the forum" (Lacan, 1932, p. 212). The structure of these disorders reflects their genesis in social relationships, their emergence within the family, and their integration into the personality. In this, what he calls the *anomalies of the family situation* and the *psychic anomaly* appear as moments and events that favor the flowering of psychopathologies. These anomalies spring up at home and in the family circle, and according to Lacan, they do not respond to the laws of heredity.

> We see, in fact, when we closely study these cases, that the notion of a hereditary transmission, so debatable in psychology, does not need to be invoked. The anamnesis always shows that the influence of the environment was exerted sufficiently to explain the transmission of the disorder.
>
> (Lacan, 1932, p. 285 [*Translated by the author*])

It was not clear at that time what this family anomaly consisted of, however, he does emphasize the presence of a psychic anomaly in the parent of the same sex as the psychotic; not as a hereditary fact but as "unconscious inter-reactions" between individuals inside a family nucleus.

In both the Seminar on *The Psychoses* carried out between 1955 and 1956 and three years later in his article *On a question prior to any possible treatment of psychosis* (Lacan, 1959), Lacan begets an interesting gap with respect to this idea of the anomaly of the family situation and a paternal imago not installed in the psychotic. This gap does not radically break the links with the writings of the 1930s, but it does show the entry of structuralism into the author's mindset. It is no longer an anomaly, nor the lack of paternal imago, but the foreclosure[1], the non-inscription of the primordial signifier of the paternal function, that would be at the heart of psychosis. Lacan calls this signifier Name-of-the-Father (from now on NotF), and its non-inscription foreclosure. The paternal signifier supports and promulgates the Law, not only in legal matters but also in ethical matters (Lacan, 1957–1958). This may be Lacan's greatest contribution to understanding the "constitutional element" of psychosis (Lacan, 1932, p. 286), which he suspected or sought as early as in his doctoral thesis. Lacan never abandoned this hypothesis, maintaining it until the end of his work in the 1970s, albeit with certain variations in what post-Lacanians call the "clinic of the Borromean knots". In fact, the concept of the NotF is preserved in the topology of the Borromean knots, as indicated in the lectures of Seminar *R.S.I.* on March 11, 1975 and April 15, 1975, where he declares it as the naming function and the fourth knot that holds together the other three registers as the NotF. Contrary to the claims of some Lacanian analysts, Lacan never forsook the concept in favor of the idea of a pluralized incarnation of the father figure formulated in the failed seminar of 1963, or even suggested that the concept should be ousted from his work or that the concept lost its original theoretical scope.

Is there a trigger mechanism (*trouble générateur*) for psychosis? What would that mechanism consist of? These seem to be two questions that haunted Lacan's mind for two decades. The signifier NotF and its foreclosure raise certain philosophical questions, both conceptual and epistemological, even anthropological. So forth, considering that I have sought to outline Lacan's search since the 1930s, a "socio-familiar" formula can be guessed at as the foundation of psychosis; that is, founded on the first forms of interaction with language and with the Other who might embody it.

The objective of this book is to situate where and how the concept signifier NotF comes from, even though it can be easily traced in Freud's work. His writings on, or at least around, the imago of the Father are based mainly on two of his cultural texts, *Totem and Taboo* and *Moses and Monotheism*, although the incidence of the Father can be foreshadowed from the beginning of his work (*e.g.*, in *The Interpretation of Dreams* or the cases of Dora and the Rat Man, but especially in that of Schreber). As J.-C. Maleval (2000) indicates, this concept of foreclosure of the signifier NotF "sinks roots" in Freud's work. The signifier NotF also, to a large extent, draws on the structural anthropology of Claude Lévi-Strauss, as I will elaborate in more detail throughout the book. This direct connection of the concept with these two authors can be inferred through a philological approach to Lacan's work, and many authors such as Maleval (2000) and E. Porge (2013) have already followed this path. However, continuing to follow it does not seem to bear fruit, so a detour is necessary, especially if what I want is to demonstrate the *logical and genealogical* stances the idea of this primordial signifier stand on. Tracing and describing them will offer an answer to the questions that will guide this book: How should one ascribe epistemological consistency to the concept of the signifier NotF? And, especially, why is it so meaningful to the understanding of psychosis?

If Freud started from a methodological individualism to account for social facts, Lacan enters through psychiatry and structural anthropology in a top-down vision towards a non-reductive individualism of psychopathology, depending on social facts[2] (independently of any hypothetical etiological underpinnings). The NotF is a starting point to propose a social ontology coming from Lacan and psychoanalysis. Social ontology in the sense of what are social facts and what they consist of, or what are facts that arise in the world of social beings endowed with language. The latter and its concepts depend on social interactions, which in turn depend on language. Social ontology seeks to understand how the social world is constructed. It's a field of philosophy interested in the questions

> about what the constituents of social reality and the relationships between them are… if there is such a thing as a limited 'social world', how is that world connected with the rest of reality, or, also, how is it possible for various individuals to act together.
>
> (Ramos and Ramírez, 2018, pp. 9–10 [*Translated by the author*])

Whilst I will clarify that this book is not directly about social ontology, it will, however, use a supported reading in this field to understand the genea-logical process of the "signifier NotF". Genealogical, in the Nietzschean–Foucauldian sense, because it involves searching for the origins and molding of a social fact, the types of belief, attitude, and jouissance imposed by the disguises of power in interpreting that fact, both in the formation of a logico-grammatically supported rationality and within collective practices over a large period of space-time. So, we can state that the concept of NotF enjoys a historico-anthropological background and is generated in the encounter between linguistic beings with intentions and propositional attitudes. Genealogical historiography, in terms of F. Nietzsche, tries to unravel from history what remains silent, addressing neglected or ignored events, or apparently anodyne or anecdotal, seeking to sustain "that which can be documented, which can actually be confirmed and has actually existed, in short, the whole, long, hard-to-decipher hieroglyphic script of man's moral past" (Nietzsche, 2008, p. 8). The paternal function within language, which Lacan wields in a declarative way, goes hand-in-hand with the power that precedes it, with the activity of naming, says Nietzsche. The power to name, speak, and occupy a place of deontic and apophantic statements is preceded by discourses and by the different positions occupied by the figures of mastery and the changes in the libidinal economy (pleasure-unpleasure, jouissance, and desire).

My proposal is logical because it is based on set theory, and more precisely, on Alain Badiou's work on ontology, *Being and Event* (Badiou, 2005). The choice to start with a logical dissertation buttressed on set theory is due, first, to the fact that it avoids directly conflicting with meaning effects. The advantage of the mathematical procedure, or of its logic in this case, is that it works in a vacuum, that is to say, it is pure formality, managing to establish a system escaping from the qualities and difficulties of the referent. Second, as Alain Badiou (2005) indicates, it brings to the fore the problem of the multiple and the one (unity) by showing that set theory is a reflection on ontology, on what *is* and is *presented.* It is the science of being qua being, being as being. For Badiou, ontology is a situation (Badiou, 2005, p. 27), and a situation is "any presented multiplicity… the place of taking-place, whatever the terms of the multiplicity in question. Every situation admits its own particular operator of the count-as-one" (Badiou, 2005, p. 24). This means that ontology is where the actions of agents who participate in a shared space are deployed, in which mutual expectations emerge in accordance with regular practices, it is an intentional activity that favors forming-into-one of any situation, whose orientation can be understood based on the history of interaction of those agents. Naming, pointing out, and acting among agents around diversified objects and inconsistent multiplicities is what makes it possible to agree on the consistency of the one. In this sense, it could be said that for Badiou the term "social ontology" would be redundant, as all ontology *is* social.

Counting as an individual depends on an operation; it is the result of an operation where a multiple, which always precedes it, begins to count-as-one. There must be a structure to the presentation so that the multiple can be counted as one. "A structure allows number to occur within the presented multiple. […] What will have been counted as one, on the bases of not having been one, turns out to be multiple" (Badiou, 2005, p. 24). Set theory facilitates naming or gathering under one designation a multiple, gathering a collection of objects into one (a whole), as defined by G. Cantor. What is expected, and this was also Lacan's bet when he tried to pass his hypotheses through the sieve of logic, is that the formalization of a concept makes it possible to draw the limits so that nothing exceeding that multiple comes to destabilize it. What is important in set theory is how the concept adheres to or can be tied to the multiple, belongs to it or is a member of it ($\in$), or is included in it ($\subset$). Its way of belonging or being included (*without being the same*) gives character to the presentation. Lacan intended not to study the speaking subject in entifying and substantializing terms, as psychology or neurosciences do today, but based on purely formal and logical thought, which does not exclude the substance. It is, as indicated by Gómez Camarena (2018), the possibility of symbolizing Imaginary data or how to connect the Imaginary with the Symbolic.

Another interest in applying set theory is that it also involves the pre-conceptual. In other words, before there is a possible concept, there is already a multiplicity that can only be presented by another multiplicity that preexists it. "The sign $\in$, unbeing of any one, determines, in a uniform manner, the presentation of 'something' as indexed to the multiple" (Badiou, 2005, p. 44). Hence, a preexistent multiplicity can be derived from the axiomatization of set theory. This is how multiplicity is formed-into-one by obeying certain inevitable and structural rules. The axiomatization of set theory was intended to maintain a logicist attitude,

> to base set theory directly on logic, i.e., either to consider set theory, and mathematics in general, as part of logic and to obtain the set-theoretical truths as logical truths, or, what turned out to be more adequate, to introduce some of the set-theoretical truths as axioms and deduce from them other set-theoretical truths by means of logic only.
>
> (Fraenkel, Bar-Hillel, and Levy, 2001, p. 17)

To begin looking at the composition of this text, in the first part of the book, "The logical dissertation: the zero symbolic value of the Name-of-the-Father", I will try to follow as rigorously as possible, standing on the logic of sets, the axiomatic necessity of an empty set for an indefinite multiple to start counting as one. For example, in the set of natural numbers, one must start from something that does not fall into a set, which we call zero, so that it can later be counted as 1. That was the intention of G. Frege and, in a similar way, of M. Heidegger, who tried to demonstrate the logical necessity of passing from the void to the thing, a logical order of arriving at a presentation of the object that stands-there. Being able to predicatively judge and know an object requires a pre-predicative movement, or a metastructure, which manages to set in motion the presentation—this, thanks to Freud's coined concept of the original repression (*Urverdrängung*).

In the second Chapter, I try to introduce language as a set, just as Lacan intended to do. One can start from the principle that a language requires a set (curly brackets {} are used to indicate one), and something that belongs to it and is included. Following linguist F. de Saussure, that set requires at least one "ordered pair", the signifiers $\{S_1\}$ and the signified $\{S_1, S_2\}$. Lacan replaces the latter, the signified, with

A, the initial letter of the big Other in French, or the battery of signifiers, the locus where the signifiers become relevant due to their ability to link propositionally. So $\{S_1, A\}$ will be the Language set, but insofar as S_1 is included in A ($S_1 \subset A$), we can simply call it {A}. The speaking subject, which Lacan designates with a crossed-out S, $, will be included and at the same time excluded in a Russell's paradox in {A}. Its permanence as a member of the {A} is neither inside nor outside. How can a $ operate if it is neither inside nor outside {A}? In Chapter 3, I seek to answer that question by establishing the original act of negation through pre-predicative judgments of the types attributional and existential (Freud, 1925). The original repression (*Urverdrängung*) takes place as an inaugural existential judgment, where the existent would be the presentation to the senses of the object and its correspondence to a state of affairs in the world, but by negating some of its idealized, desired, and fantasized traits. This is because negation settles a "not belonging to" property of the legality of sets ($\alpha \notin \beta$). It implies what Lacan calls the Thing (*das Ding*), not just as some sort of pre-predicative judgment but as an alienating and dialectic stance; the Thing is the lost Real[3] object, necessary for the principle of reality to overcome.

In a second moment, the act of naming takes on its importance; only a multiple can begin to count-as-one, but starting from an initial void, which we can call {ø}. The name of this multiple is what favors suturing it to Language (*langage*), turning it into the noun-phrase of a proposition. Then, negating and being named with a proper name (to be later able to name) come as potentialities for the uses of language (*langue*) and the process of subjectivization. This means that the subject counts as multiple-one, but without being co-opted by the signifiers of the Other.

In Chapter 4, I seek to outline the pre-existence of a metastructure for any presentation. Badiou (2005) suggests that a metastructure "gathers together all the sub-compositions of internal multiples, all the inclusions" (p. 83). The NotF would be that metastructure, as the first body of the signifier. The NotF is that first body schema or form that, in psychosis, for Lacan, finds itself rejected or—to use the term he uses—foreclosed (*verworfen*). If we follow the anthropologists M. Mauss and C. Lévi-Strauss, we find that the minimal operations of language require an opposition between signifiers, an operation that is very illustrative in languages where there is a signifier with antithetical signifieds. The case of the signifier "mana", in certain parts of Asia, indicates a wide range of referents; this is, it would have a *zero symbolic value*, acting almost as {ø} for the signified, which any element can come to belong to. The signifier NotF would be of the type of zero symbolic value signifiers; many names can come to occupy its place both as designator and referent. However, despite the zero symbolic value enjoyed by a first body of signifier such as NotF, it does not represent lack. How can lack be a member of any set, especially {A}? So, we have a signifier of lack, S(A̸), and a signifier of zero symbolic value that provide metastructure and corporeality to any presentation.

To conclude this first part, in Chapter 5, I include the second necessary operation in order to enter language, after we saw in Chapter 3 how the axiom of the empty set indicated that there exists a set such as null element is a member of it. The second operation facilitating the emergence of S(A̸), according to Lacan, depends on an act of privation. Something must be extracted from the set of multiples, something must act as agent. This is what Freud called castration. This castration will be of an Imaginary object ($-\varphi$) but generating a lack in the Symbolic (Φ)—Lacan called it the phallic signifier—and expelling an object into the Real (object petit *a*). We'll see why precisely this signifier is *phallic*.

Lacan sought to formalize the encounter of the family triangle as a structuring instance, where the Oedipus complex leaves as a result this castration or extraction of the object *a* (a generic term to designate any Freudian drive or instinctual object). This castration is constitutive and is precisely what is not carried out in psychosis due to the non-inscription of the signifier NotF (Lacan, 1959). If the signifier Φ and NotF are not inscribed in $\{A\}$, the lack $S(\not{A})$ comes to lack or is negated, $\neg S(\not{A})$, the object *a* is not extracted, resulting in a psychotic structure. I will take this matter more into detail in the text.

In the second part of the book, "A genealogy of *The Father* and the death of the Father: a quest through jouissance and Modernity", I start with a historiographical and genealogical work on the structural bases of the Father. Patriarchy and then monotheism bring a certain number of regulations and parameters for male/female relationships and sexuality, revealing an impasse in this relationship. Gerda Lerner (1986) suggests how the mythology of ancient Mesopotamian civilizations demonstrates the transforming and dynamic relationships of language, or the relationships between signifier and signified. For instance, procreation and origins enjoyed mythical referents that went from spontaneous female fertility to "conscious and reasoned" sexual encounters. Up until a certain epoch, the myths of procreation were no longer just a confirmation of spontaneous origin, but a symbolic and abstract enactment that had to overcome all kinds of tests and feats to happen. For Lerner, this opens the way to monotheism, to the One-God, the infinite multiple under one name of an infinite and impossible set. What this multiple and its attribution of will and desire implies, however, is a first form of recognition of the Hebrew God towards man, when on Mount Sinai Yahwe bequeathed Moses the tablets of the ten commandments. Lacan follows: "The underlying prelude of those commandments is the *You are* that appoints you as *I*" (Lacan, 1968–1969, p. 80). The introduction of the Law, represented in that table of the Ten Commandments, also plays a preponderant role in the way in which speech is articulated. The Commandments, "in their indestructible character... prove to be the very laws of speech [*parole*]..." (Lacan, 1959–1960, p. 174). They are the rules for organizing subsets in order to operate with all sorts of multiples; of course, they are not axiomatic rules but deontic (also conative) and apophantic operators.

In Chapter 7, that god of monotheism and the Old Testament is an authoritarian god who does not forgive enemies, who punishes, and who demands blood and vengeance. In the genocides apparently committed in his name, we deduce the presence of what Lacan calls jouissance. How is this unchained jouissance that prevents the formation of a culture regulated? The Father God of the Law appears as a normative entity that fulfills a "sublimatory function", favoring a certain "apprehension of reality as such" and a "normalization of desire" (Lacan, 1959–1960,

p. 181). This Real father, who is a dead, mythical, structural father, is the agent of castration, the establisher of language as the locus of locutionary and subjective assumptions.

In Chapter 8, I explore the thesis put forward by Littlewood and Dein (2013) on the origins of psychosis in the rise of Modernity and individualism. This thesis is indebted to Georges Devereux. Certain philosophico-religious positions and dogmas, such as those of Augustine of Hippo and, later in the 17th century, Francis Bacon and René Descartes, merged with the new dogmas of Protestantism coming from the 16th century. This favored the emergence of the *self* and of self-awareness; the individual as a multiple of the collective now counts as an indivisible one. A decisive and anthropological mutation forged a new metaphysics of *ontos*.

Chapter 9 intends to investigate in more detail how this mutation occurs within the family, or more precisely, the Father and his name and the role they play. The bet of Emile Durkheim and Lacan in *Les complexes familiaux dans la formation de l'individu* (1938) is to deem Modernity and individualism as precursors of a new type of family conformation: the conjugal family. This is a type of family based on what Durkheim called the "law of family contraction", which, according to him, led to an almost deficient family arrangement. It would be problematic since it would neutralize the role of the *pater familias*, the figure of the great Patriarch, decimating his imago. In addition, it would sharpen individualism, family breakdown, anomie, and suicide (Zafiropoulos, 2002). However, this reading of Durkheim will be widely refuted and questioned by other historical studies that suggest that the conjugal and reduced family was the common denominator throughout the Middle Ages, and even before. This figure of the great Patriarch, the father of the stem and extensive family, would be rather rare, closer to a fantasy, and limited to certain noble families. Lacan would end up detouring from this idea of a law of family contraction, even moving away from Durkheim. For Lacan, it will no longer be a question of a decline of the father's imago, not even of the flesh-and-blood father's power, incarnated in any man (or woman). At this moment, the NotF makes its entry into the work of Lacan, more precisely in his article *Le mythe individuel du névrosé* (1953), a reinterpretation of Rat Man's case contrasted with Schreber's. Now, however, the father will gain symbolic value, insofar as that Father signifier belongs to the Real, *i.e.*, an impossible one.

Chapter 10 takes up the works of fiction from theater and cinema to portray the way in which the century of Revolutions and the centuries of Postmodernism give way to a reliable example of the figure of the Imaginary father and its Symbolic place. The theater of Paul Claudel, with the Coûfontaine trilogy, introduced by Lacan in his Seminar *Transference*, and the cinema of the Coen brothers, with what I call the "father trilogy", serve as illustrations of the way in which the figure of the father is depicted in a world that is transformed due to the loss of references and the exacerbation of individualism. The Coen brothers' trilogy has the structure of a myth as I'll try to demonstrate.

The third and final part, "A socio-ontological appraisal of psychosis", begins with John Searle's contributions to the theory of social ontology. He introduces status function declarations (SFD) as utterances of the performative type. His goal is to explain how SFD bear social facts when the collective recognizes them as such and endows them with deontic power. If they fit under a general formula like "X counts as Y in C", with C being the context, SFD would provide the institutional reality.

However, Searle's formula does not consider which of these counts do not enter the count. This is the eventful site, which, according to Badiou, encompasses the unpresented elements of the presentation. In this sense, Searle's "X counts as Y in C" indicates that C is not just anything, that it is a C loaded with history and possibilities of historicization and reinterpretation, composed of elements presented and unpresented, revealed and veiled. This is what constitutes the ontological richness of the eventful site. C can count as one or a series of historizable events. For C to be the eventfulness of a multiple, a naming and interpretative intervention must be carried out by speaking beings that authorize "X *to count* as Y in C". At this point, the algebra of Lacan's discourses enters the scene, since the elements that compose it, \$, S_1, S_2, and *a* suggest the configuration of subsets that can be organized according to some configuration and minimum laws. Within them, the subset of the Master's discourse represents the most prominent and widespread—in the West at least—form of accommodation of individuals with respect to the Other, desire, and truth. These loci of discourse make it easier to reference the assumed subject-position as the starting point of eventfulness. However that Master is not necessarily a supernatural figure, much less natural; that master is in Modernity the *self* or whomever speaks as I (*Je*) and who considers itself legitimate to speak. The NotF attributes corporeality to a S_1 to begin the count of all the subsets inside {A}. I'll take a brief detour into Schreber's *Memoirs* and Lacan's thesis case, Aimée, to illustrate this.

Chapter 12 focuses on an idea launched by Lacan in *L'étourdit* of 1972, where he asserts that the psychoanalyst who works with the speech of his analysands has to deal at times with the "outside-discourse of psychosis". This is outside of the ways in which discourse represents both a background and a network of meanings, and also locutionary and deontic assumed positions. Unable to adopt a clear-cut position inside any of the possible discourses regarding the *plus-de-jouir* (both as loss and surplus of that loss).

Can psychosis be conceived outside of any decompensation or onset requiring hospitalization? The proposal of untriggered psychosis or prepsychosis (Lacan, 1955–1956, p. 251) suggests a type of pre-onset psychosis that never seems to be triggered, hence the idea of a psychotic structure that roots at a certain point in life. Thus, for what remains of the book, a fundamental question emerges: How does one diagnose psychosis outside of any obvious observable phenomenon of it, *i.e.*, when there is no presence of delusions, hallucinations, negative symptoms, or disorganization of thought? The responses in the field of Lacanian psychoanalysis have been many and diverse. The key point that the course of this entire dissertation has led us to is that the assumption of a subject-position with respect to a discourse did not occur. By this we mean the way in which the subject deals with the loss or surplus of enjoyment. However precisely if no loss happened, how does a subject manage without it? Several cases are presented in this chapter and contrasted.

Finally, following the latter questions, Chapter 13 hints at the idea that perhaps it is not through the classical, medical way of diagnosing that we will understand psychosis. The lists of clinical signs and criteria do not capture the singularities of the psychotic structure. Another type of reading and approach may be more beneficial for studying and treating psychosis. The position of a socio-ontological account of psychosis acknowledges those singularities that inscribe the subject in a way of apprehending reality standing on discourse. But how does the psychotic manage to get by if it finds itself outside of discourse? If we start from the lack of lack, $\neg S(\cancel{A})$, where the non-extraction of object *a* lies, this *plus-de-jouir* cannot really be located in any of the positions that the Lacanian algebra of discourses allows, or in any case, it is something that seems problematic for the psychotic. In a presentation of a case study, I will show the original way in which a subject manages to operate with that lack of lack and with object *a* inside a reformulation of the Master's and Science's discourses. The nonmainstream body modifications in which he undertakes a life project combine the possibilities of self-therapeutics and of making up for the absence of NotF and castration (non-extraction of object *a*).

Notes

1 In English, to foreclose is to shut out, exclude, or preclude. In the legal sense, it means to take possession by force or by injunction of some good or property. In French, there is a similar meaning; however, Lacan seems to take it both from the legal world, as something definitely precluded, and from Damourette and Pichons' linguistics. For the latter, foreclosure is one of the forms of negation in the French language. For negating, usually two terms are used: *ne* and a second one that can vary, *pas*, *guère*, *rien*, *jamais*, etc., which "applies to facts that the speaker does not consider to be part of reality. These facts are in some way foreclosed, so we give this second term of negation the name of foreclosure" (Damourette and Pichon, 1928, pp. 242–243; Maleval, 2000).

2 By fact, I don't mean a concrete, observable, or material event; I mean a fact more in the sense of the constituent ordering of the "social world," *i.e.*, for Lacan, the signifier, thus speech and discourse. This is a concept closer to what Wittgenstein called *Sachverhalt* ("atomic fact"), and thus more of a logical operator than an empirical one.

3 To distinguish them from their ordinary usage, I capitalize the terms Real, Symbolic, and Imaginary. I assume that the reader has a basic understanding of Lacan's three registers of reality, which he developed throughout his work. Regarding the Real, Lacan indicates in the conference *La troisième*, from 1974, that the Real is what does not work, that is, what keeps repeating itself so as to hinder this progress, the impossible of a logical modality that keeps failing to be written down. Thus, it is that which cannot be understood nor reduced to a form of re-presentation, which resists symbolization. The Real can be thought of in relation to the Symbolic and the Imaginary as that which of the latter two is not graspable, which remains as pure impasse, a structural impossibility due to the implementation of these two registers.

Part 1

The logical dissertation

The zero symbolic value of the Name-of-the-Father

1

Nought as a non-identical identity and the empty set {ø}

Inferring the Thing

> Es ist ja Bejahung der Existenz nichts Anderes als Verneinung der Nullzahl[1].
>
> (G. Frege, 1884, §53)

1.1. From nought to one

Lacan argues that the nought value is a logical prerequisite for the existence of one. In order to count, we must start with the inexistent. For him, logic is the "art of producing a necessity[2] of discourse", where necessity is not something that is already there, but rather something that is produced through the act of discourse.

In the Seminar...*or Worse*, he writes: "already it is by no means sure that something is not reflected in, or does not contain the beginnings of [*l'amorce*], the necessity that is at issue in the precondition of animal existence" (Lacan, 1971–1972, pp. 38–39). Lacan's idea of inexistence is not the same as nothingness. Inexistence is a supposition that is necessary for the production of necessity[3]. To prove this supposition, Lacan argues that inexistence is preliminary to necessity. In the case of the symptom, what is inexistent is the truth that presupposes it. The second proof of the supposition of inexistence is the jouissance that lies behind the automatism of repetition in the symptom. The symptom, for psychoanalysis, is entrenched in the discursive necessity of truth and jouissance. It configures in analysis as a knot of signifiers confining truth and made of repetition.

However, Lacan clarifies that

> [i]t is neither through jouissance nor through truth that inexistence assumes a status, that it may inexist, in other words that it may come to the symbol that designates it as inexistence, and which, for its part, does indeed exist. As you know, this is a number that is generally designated as nought.
>
> (Lacan, 1971–1972, p. 40)

Inexistence can be expressed as a number, a natural number, more precisely the number 0. However, 0 is not nothingness, because it is a concept and therefore counts as something. It is the foundation for the existence of the natural numbers, including

DOI: 10.4324/9781032663616-3

1 and all subsequent natural numbers. According to Gottlob Frege, 0 is the number that falls under the set "not identical with itself" (Frege, 1960, §74). Identity and equivalence are not the same thing. Since there is no object that can belong to that set, the only "element" that could enter is 0 as a pure signifier. This is because 0 is the only singleton set where no object falls. A singleton is a set with only one element.

For an entity to have the value of one, it must vanish qua multiplicity. Following Frege in his *Die Grundlagen der Arithmetik* (Frege, 1960), we can argue that the concept of number, qua its use, starts from an inexistent, under which no object falls. Frege indicates that a number is identical with whatever is substitutable with it in a given proposition. Then, everything from that set belongs to another set; that is, the elements of α can be replaced by those of β while maintaining their extensionality and equivalence, $\alpha \in \beta$.

Frege's purpose is to determine how numbers are given, forasmuch as it is not something that counts as an ontological reality, "since it is only in the context of a proposition that words have any meaning, our problem becomes this: to define the sense of a proposition in which a number word occurs" (Frege, 1960, §62). The same concept of number can be used for a variety of objects because we can make judgments that express our recognition of an object identical with or belonging ($\in$), by means of certain properties (identity, substitutability, or a pattern of inferences that requires a doxastic commitment) to a given set (Brandom, 1994). In the set of "objects that fall under the Number *n*", the only thing required is for it to be able to establish a judgment-content that can be transformed into an identity, forging a pre-established relation-judgment. For example, in the case of the natural number, it must be possible to correlate one-to-one the objects that fall under the concept *F* with those that fall under the concept that follows it, *G*. Just as every object that falls into the concept *F* must be equal to all objects in the set "equal to concept *F*".

> My definition is therefore as follows:
> the number which belongs to the concept *F* is the extension of the concept 'equal to the concept *F*'.
>
> (Frege, 1960, §69)

The extensionality of the natural number implies substitutability without loss of truth value. However, the fact that the substitution of the concepts *F* and *G* maintains the truth value does not necessarily imply that both are identical; it can simply be said that one is wider than the other. For instance, if under set *F* fall all the men of New York City and under set *G* fall all the human beings with chromosomes xx who live in the largest city in the U.S., they both hold the same truth, but *G* is wider than *F*, and, of course, they are not identical. Any object that falls in the set *F* and in set *G* will be correlated by a term-to-term relationship that Frege calls *Gleichzablig*, translated as equinumerosity. The objects in both sets will be the same, even if their *designations* are not. This allows us to say that, although the set *F* is not identical with the set *G*, they are equivalent in terms of their referents. Then, if we move to the concept of natural number, we can say that the number *n* that belongs to the set *F* is the extension of the set "equal to the concept *F*". Based on the latter premise, Frege sustains in §72 that

> "*n* is a Number"
> is to mean the same as the expression
> "there exists a concept such that *n* is the Number which belongs to it".

In §74 he establishes that nought is equivalent to the concept "not identical with itself" since no object can fall under it, and because everything is considered identical with itself, if there is no object nought cannot be identical with itself and with an object to which it could be contrasted. Later in §76 he details the logic of the succession of natural numbers, and this point is key in Frege's dissertation since it indicates that the logic of the natural numbers or being a number depends on something being one or counting as one, which indicates that before there was one, there was not, or it was an inconsistent multiplicity that did not count. Frege hints that between two adjacent members of natural numbers stands a necessary relation: if a number *n* belongs to the set *F* such that an object *x* falls in that set, then the number that belongs to the set "falls under *F* but is not identical with *x*" must be *m*. However, this still doesn't indicate how to go from 0 to 1.

To prove this succession, Frege starts from a set he names "identical with 0", in which, in principle, no object falls, therefore only 0 belongs to it, as a signifier. Now, which is the *n* equinumerous to the concept "identical with 0"? It will be the number that maintains the one-to-one relationship, starting with 0, but not being 0, and whose sequence will respond to (n+1). The number 1, then, as counterintuitive as it may seem, belongs to the set "identical with 0", because in this set *at least one* object falls, 0. Following the logical premise of §76, the number that falls under the concept "identical with 0 but is not a null object" is 1. Therefore, the number that follows 0 in the series of natural numbers is 1. This could also be read as: There is an empty concept ø in which no object falls, such that the number belonging to ø is 0, and the following number that belongs to the concept "falling under ø but not identical with 0" is 1 (Frege, §76). *This means that 0 is structurally necessary for there to be 1* (nought being the only "element" part of the empty set identical and different from itself) (Frege, §77). The empty set {ø} is the only subset of all sets, universally included. The moment something arises in that set, it can start to be counted, but it will no longer be an empty set. "Clearly, the equinumerosity of the concept under which no object falls, in the capacity of inexistence, is always equal to itself" (Lacan, 1971–1972, p. 46).

1.2. The Thing and the presentation of the inconsistent

The basic axioms of set theory assume that, in order to have a set as a collection of elements, something has to count-as-one, belong to, or be included in the set (without belonging and including being exactly the same thing). Therefore, in an empty set, nothing belongs to it or is included, calling into question its quality as a set. Thus, something must fall under the concept of one, hold an identity with the concept of 0, but not be a null object. There must be an apprehensible presentation as one or at least as a consistent multiple, precisely ignoring, or not taking into account, the inconsistency of the multiple. "Multiple is said of a presentation, in that it is retroactively apprehended as non-one as soon as being-one is a result" (Badiou, 2005, p. 25). Exactly that inconsistency is what the metastructure frames, at the same time that which is veiled by the presentation, that is, the inexistent, on the one hand, and the void, on the other. The void is the original inconsistency that is subtracted from the count, as Alain Badiou (2005) tells us, which means that "the unpresentable is presented, as a subtractive term of the presentation of presentation. Or: a multiple is, which is not under the Idea of the multiple" (Badiou, 2005, pp. 67–68). Or, continues Badiou, as a multiple that cannot be thought of under the concept of multiple, or—to make the argument even clearer—a being that can be named but whose existence is totally uncertain even though we can suppose it. The one arises as an effect of the count and of the structure that frames it, as a count-as-one or structure of the *nominal seal* of the multiple, and at the same time as the *effect of one*, "whose fictive being is maintained solely by the structural retroaction in which it is considered" (Badiou, 2005, p. 90).

In the Seminar on *The Ethics of Psychoanalysis*, Lacan had already laid out how an object begins to count as an object, as one, in its process from thing to signifying function. Following Martin Heidegger, he applies the example of a vase (although Heidegger speaks of a jug, for effects, both are a vessel or container); what characterizes it as a thing is the fact that it starts from the void, "in its signifying function is that in which in its incarnated form characterizes the vase as such. It creates the void and thereby introduces the possibility of filling it" (Lacan, 1959–1960, p. 120). It is in this form entrenched in the void and the possibility of filling it that, for Lacan, a dialectic is introduced into the world, that of the empty and the full.

Heidegger, from whom Badiou derived a good part of his dissertation, also seeks to locate the passage from nought to one as the passage from the void to the thing and then to the object. This is the logical order of the presentation, an inevitable order. For Heidegger, a jug, for example, is an *object* insofar as we *re*-present it to ourselves, either as a perception or a memory, or as that which becomes the object of a representation. However, what makes the jug a thing, or where does the thinghood of the jug reside? "Standing-on-its-own seemed to characterize the jug as a thing", which makes it an object, but that objectivity of the object and the objectivity of the standing-on-its-own does not indicate its thinghood. The material of which the jug is made also tells us nothing about what it makes of a thing, thing. What makes the jug a thing is that it is a container, a vessel, capable of embracing the void,

> the empty is what holds in the vessel. The empty, this nothing in the jug, is what the jug is as a holding vessel. [...] The thinghood of the vessel by no means rests in the materials of which it consists, but instead in the emptiness that holds.
>
> (Heidegger, 2012, pp. 7–8)

When the potter fashions the jug, it is in order to mold a shape with the clay, but it is not exactly the clay that is shaped, it is the void that is molded, and the entire manufacturing process consists of that molding. The thinghood of the thing must remain hidden as the *thing* is not presented as *a* thing in its essence. In this matter, the thinghood cannot access thought or language, nor presentation. That is to say, the thinghood of the thing is basically what is elusive, ineffable, and what vanishes from the presentation.

Lacan borrows and differentiates the concept of thing, in German *Ding*, from another word that is usually also translated as thing from that language, *Sache*. He employs the former to approach the moral law as what covers the Real, precisely where *das Ding* appears as a substrate of the Real. *Ding* is used in a legal sense as the passage to the Symbolic order of a conflict between people, which consists of a legal proceeding. In Latin, the closest word is "res", which relates to "causa", the cause, or an affair. The old High Germanic word *thing* or *dinc*, meaning gathering, became a name for an affair that committed the people to a gathering for a negotiation. "The wrapping and the presentation of the concrete", that is, the symbolization of tension or matter of discussion between speaking beings. However, the word *Sache* is used in a different way, more in an abstract manner or one which does not include any materiality. For example, when one says of someone that "he knows how to do his things", in German one employs *Sache* rather than *Ding*; in this, *Sache* is a product or result of human action governed by language, hence *Sache* and *Wort* (word) are related, especially in Freud's paper *The Unconscious* where he contrasts the concept of *Sachevorstellung* and *Wortvorstellung*; but *das Ding* is not. The *Ding* only becomes allusive to the extent that it becomes a word, rather it is what remains isolated in the presentation, in the *Vorstellung* and its re-presentation (*Darstellung*), as pure symbolic abstract processing. The presentation figures as an intermediary between *perceptum* and *percipiens*, "between the glove and the hand", and is governed by the pleasure principle and the impulse to find again, to reencounter a lost object, which was never an actual part of any presentation at all but a fantasy. The succession of re-presentations (*Darstellung*), by the intermediary of the signifier, presented again, follows the basic mechanisms of the unconscious and thought process (condensation and displacement), "the small curds of representation, that is to say, something which has the same structure as the signifier" (Lacan, 1959–1960, p. 61).

> Right at the beginning of the organization of the world in the psyche, both logically and chronically, *das Ding* is something that presents and isolates itself as the strange feature around which the whole movement of the *Vorstellung* turns—a *Vorstellung* that Freud shows us is governed by a regulatory principle, the so-called pleasure principle, which is tied to the functioning of the neuronic apparatus. And it is around *das Ding* that the whole adaptive development revolves, a development that is so specific to man insofar as the symbolic process reveals itself to be inextricably woven into it.
>
> (Lacan, 1959–1960, p. 57)

According to this quote, one can infer the Thing as something that appears as an "in-between-three", as the elusive mediation in order to achieve the (necessary) logical passage of the void to the inexistent and, finally, to the signifying (conceptual) re-presentation of the object, which I have been insinuating. Lacan states that the Thing is "the beyond-of-the-signified. It is as a function [...] and of an emotional relationship to it that the subject keeps its distance and is constituted in a kind of relationship characterized by primary affect, prior to any repression" (Lacan, 1959–1960, p. 54). Hence, the Thing is what is alien to me at the same time that it is the most intimate, at my core, the *ex-timate*. It stands as a prehistoric Other, which ensures a form of total pleasure, impossible in its own ineffability and signifying inapprehensibility. The Thing is "that which in the [R]eal suffers from the signifier" (Lacan, 1959–1960, p. 125).

1.3. The Thing: the unpresented transgression of the law

Following Freud's work, the concept of *thing* (*das Ding*) would prefigure a specific pre-predicative judgment (Husserl, 1973, §§ 8–9), tied to attribution and existence judgments (see Chapter 3). The phenomenological point of view, which Badiou implicitly exposes in his logical procedure, involves describing how what is perceived arrives at and is apprehended by consciousness. The way of constituting the objects through an assimilation of the presentation (*Vorstellung*); presentation is the way in which cognition is produced before any *perceptum*. For Edmund Husserl, who is considered the creator of the phenomenological method, consciousness is the fundamental condition of the "constitution" of objects. The constitution is therefore a process that will allow us to grasp through our senses the objects in our environment—objects in front of us—through our sight, touch, hearing, etc. For him, for example, every judgment of a presentation depends on a horizon of possibilities that is given in advance, there is a passive pre-given background of sense experiences that favor knowing and judging the object. Everything that exhibits to the senses as a presented object enjoys a pre-given degree of familiarity, of trustworthiness.

Das Ding, in Freud's *Project for a Scientific Psychology*, indicates the presence of an-other, the fellow being (*Nebenmensch*), as necessary for predicative judgments to come into operation (Freud, 1895). The proximity of the fellow being ensures an objective horizon of the infant's perceptions. The Other appears, in principle, for the baby, as an object, first of satisfaction, then of hostility, but also as the main form of "helping power" and horizon of meaning (figure-ground). Coming to cognize and predicatively judge is only going to be possible with the intermediation of the Other. For instance, body movements are learned from the observation of the other and its imitation; if someone moves an arm in a certain way, the toddler will try to do the same and will try to associate it with memory impressions of their previous movements. In this process, the Other, representing a complex, "falls apart into two components, of which one makes an impression by its constant structure and stays together as a thing [*als Ding*], while the other can be understood by the activity of memory—that is, can be traced back to information from [the subject's] own body" (Freud, 1895, p. 331). Let's recall that a "complex" is the fixation of developing imagos and presentation apprehensions of identifications, whose constitution is enabled by the image of a parental figure.

Now, Lacan interprets the apprehension of reality as a twofold event, what persists in memory of the impressions of the other, and something else. There is a differentiation in the approach to the perceptive judgment of the object, in the sense that something inside ends up appearing on the outside as a presentation. In an outside that "has nothing to do with that reality in which the subject will subsequently have to locate the *Qualitätszeichen* [qualitative characteristic]" (Lacan, 1959–1960, p. 52) of the presentation of reality. He suggests that something sifts and sorts out the presentation of objects, or "deals with selected bits of reality" (Lacan, 1959–1960, p. 47). He goes a step further in regard to Freud's (or even Husserl's) reading of the pre-predicative judgment as the Thing. The Thing is more (or less?) than that; it seems to be what isolates itself in the Other as alienating (*Fremde*), an unpresented aspect of the Other that indicates the world of desires and expectations, a dialectic in which the baby becomes implicated and that presents to it what the object covers. So, it is some alterity of the Other that presents as alienating and disquieting for the child. Not only that, Lacan's reading is that this first external object is around which the perceptual and re-presentative orientation of the subject is situated.

However, Lacan will imply that the Thing is *also* the lost object that was experienced as satisfying, or the first form of satisfaction (the pleasure principle), ergo, the mother. "[T]he Sovereign Good, which is *das Ding*, which is the mother, is also the object of incest, is a forbidden good, and... there is no other good" (Lacan, 1959–1960, p. 70). So, it combines pleasure–unpleasure, and privation in the guise of the maternal libidinal object. This is what the Thing represents, and it is a cover-up for the transgression of the fundamental law: the prohibition of incest. Lacan stresses that the pleasure principle is not limited to a purely biological or physiological experience that is totally self-centered. Rather, it implies the Other (in its encompassing horizon of legality and meaning) as an unpresented fact that is essential to the apprehension of a presentation. The Freudian concept of *Vorstellungsrepräsentanz* (representative of the presentation) is what in the unconscious re-presents the presentation as a sign in its function of apprehension—

> of the way in which every (re)presentation is represented insofar as it evokes the good that *das Ding* brings with it. [...] Everything that qualifies (re)presentations in the order of the good is caught up in refraction, in the atomized structure that the system of the unconscious facilitations imposes, in the complex mechanism of a signifying system of elements. It is only in that way that the subject relates to that which presents itself on the horizon as his good.
>
> (Lacan, 1959–1960, pp. 71–72)

Freud's question is, what of that Thing can be rediscovered in the perception of reality?

> It is now no longer a question of whether what has been perceived (a thing) shall be taken into the ego or not, but of whether something which is in the ego as a presentation can be rediscovered in perception (reality) as well.
>
> (Freud, 1925, p. 237)

The Thing can appear in any possible perception, and every perception implies the Thing and the affective value it contains at the moment of apprehension. Freud's bet is that this jump from the void to a thing, both alienating and harmonizing, will set up the subsequent judicative encounters with the metonymic series of objects that the baby will encounter and represent in a lifetime. The passage of this unpresentable Thing, settled in the void, towards the formation of the first signifier (S_1) is an important leap that depends on the original repression (*Urverdrängung*). I'll come back to this matter in the third chapter. This passage is essential to the formation of reality for any individual. For Freud, it is not about finding the factual correspondence between the object and our mental representation of it, or between *Wahrnehmung* and *Bewusstsein*, but about rediscovering what our desire captured as a source of satisfaction, *framed by the signifying structure*. Reality-testing aims to identify which aspect of the lost Thing can be found again in any perception. Reality perception can never find its pleasure coordinates on its own; rather, it is necessary to seek "the optimum tension; below that there is neither perception nor effort" (Lacan, 1959–1960, p. 52). This indicates that something of the order of the hallucinatory, of what we expect and wish for, is necessary for the world of perception to be organized. "The world of perception is represented by Freud as dependent on that fundamental hallucination without which there would be no attention attainable" (Lacan, 1959–1960, p. 53).

Notes

1 "Affirmation of existence is nothing but negation of the number nought".
2 In Aristotle's *Prior Analytics*, necessity is what appears as unavoidable in the deduction of certain premises. So, it shows as that which is entailed from a series of organized premises posing certain antecedents and that must lead to a unique and impending conclusion. "[A] syllogism is discourse (*logos*) in which, certain things being stated, something other than what is stated follows of necessity from their being so. I mean by the last phrase that they produce the consequence, and by this, that no further term is required from without in order to make the consequence necessary. I call a perfect syllogism which needs nothing other than what has been stated to make plain what necessarily follows" (Aristotle, 1952, p. 39: 24b19–26).
3 Even though one might wonder where one should place logical necessity in cultures where the concept of number does not exist, for example, consider the case of the indigenous people of the Brazilian Amazon, the Pirahã. Their language has been widely studied and debated in academic linguistic circles after linguist Daniel Everett lived with them for years and stated that their language did not possess recursion, subordinate clauses, or words for numbers or colors. Everett indicates that there is no number because there is no need for numbers within their cultural practices. Where do we place the logical need for discourse in them? Although there is no need for numbers, there is the idea of that which is present and that which is not, of the one or the multiple that forms-into-one, and of that which is inexistent or that which does not present itself.

2

The inconsistency of the Language set and the divided subject

2.1. The ordered pair of language and the uncertainty of the Other

The logic of sets that I have been using can help us to understand not only ontology, or the equivalence between ontology and mathematics that authors like Badiou have shown, but also how to think about language using the same logic of sets. For Lacan, language can be considered within set theory because language and discourse are made up of chains of signifiers that follow certain axioms. Thus, we can start with an "ordered pair", which is the relationship of a signifier S′ with another signifier S″, S′-S″. Following Lacan's classic and repeated dictum of what a signifier means according to its mode of use: *it is what represents a subject for another signifier*, we can have a minimal ordered pair for language (*langue*). He initially represents it as a set of two elements, which are themselves two subsets: that of the signifier $\{S_1\}$ and that of the signified $\{S_1, S_2\}$ (Lacan will simply call this last subset S_2, where $S_2 \in S_2$ and the signified is the product of the propositional chaining of various signifiers). By extension we can write the Language as set A: $\{ø, \{S_1\}, \{S_1, S_2\}\}$ or, for short, A: $\{\{S_1\}, \{S_2\}\}$. Another way in which Lacan designates S_2 is precisely as A, the big Other, the locus and treasure trove of signifiers, it can then also be written as A: $\{ø, \{S_1\}, \{A\}\}$, where $A \in \{A\}$ ("A belongs to or is a member of set A"). The Other is a place where all signifiers are linked together to form meanings propositionally. Lacan postulates that this big Other (with an initial capital A in French) is the radical other that constitutes and pre-exists us. It is the warrant of truth, the locus of the code, of signifiers, and ultimately the wall of language and institutionality. The big Other plays a role as a third party in any form of exchange where utterances and actions are legitimized and sustained, but it is especially the locus that is addressed in any psychoanalysis as the space where the unconscious resides.

We can pose A as the set of all linked signifiers that contains itself. However, Lacan demonstrates that this A, as an element of itself, cannot be counted as an element of itself, $A \notin A$. It falls into Russell's paradox, *i.e.*, being trapped inside and outside the set. For example, the set of all sets contains itself as an element of

DOI: 10.4324/9781032663616-4

the set. And what about the set of all sets that are not members of themselves? The latter means falling into a paradox or antinomy.

Suppose that I want to organize my library with two bookshelves: on shelf A are all the books that do not contain or reference themselves, and on shelf B are those that do reference themselves. Next, I want to make a catalog for each shelf of the books available on it. However, a problem arises, especially with the catalog of shelf A. Since this catalog must be referenced as being part of the list of books on shelf A and it is part of that shelf, it could not be placed on that shelf because self-referential books do not go there. So, it would have to go on shelf B, but since it is not a book belonging to that shelf it cannot reference itself as being part of shelf A, and since it does not self-reference, it could not go either on shelf B. This creates a paradox. Where should one place the catalog for shelf A?

Lacan relies on another ordered pair: S, as a signifier, and A as an Other signifier, a set of two elements, which also are sets themselves. Let's call it set A or $(S \rightarrow A)$, read as *S then A*. If A, moreover, as already indicated, is also the big Other, a treasure trove of signifiers, how should one posit it as a signifier of a relationship the same signifier that intervenes in this relationship? Can A, which designates this set, be the same A that is part of its intrinsic property as a set, A be a member of $\{A\}$?

> We are going to have a series of circles... and an indefinite repetition of the S, without ever being able to stop the backward movement, if I may say so, of the A. [...]
>
> That the big A as such has in it this flaw which is due to the fact that one cannot know what it contains, if not its own signifier, here is a decisive question where what is there is revealed as the flaw of knowledge. Insofar as it is at the locus of the Other that the possibility of the subject is suspended as it is formulated, it is most important to know that what would guarantee it, namely the place of truth, is itself a faulty place.
>
> (Lacan, 1968–1969, pp. 58–59 [*Translated by the author*])

However, this still doesn't demonstrate the ambiguity of A and its lack through the sole logical justification. Let's remember extensionality, that is, any set X can be replaced by a set Y as long as its properties and truth conditions are maintained. Then $A \in \{A\}$ could be replaced by $S_1, S_2, S_3 \in \{S_1, S_2, S_3\}$, each signifier of the treasure trove of signifiers would belong in a tautology to itself, the signifier beach is beach, the signifier dog is dog. In that totalizing and self-contained figure of A, only redundancy and periphrasis would fit. However, the semantic property of the signifier is that it does not refer to itself, but to other signifiers. For this reason, it does not meet the conditions of a self-referential set, since A includes elements that would not be elements of themselves, that is, other signifiers. So, we should say that $A \notin \{A\}$ ("A is not a member of set A"), therefore, A should be part of the subset of elements that do not contain themselves, however, that subset is A itself. And we have already said that A could not contain itself. We then fall into Russell's paradox. This paradox extends to the relationship between the signifier and the signified: they cannot be thought of as included in the other, nor as excluded from each other.

So, returning to Lacan's definition of a signifier as that which represents the subject for another signifier, where does one locate the speaking subject in relation to set A? Is the subject, as Lacan writes it \$ (a crossed-out S), outside or inside the set? Is the \$ a property of the elements, that is, of S_1 and of A, or a subset of A? Lacan gives clues to suppose that \$ is a subset of A, this is, included in A: $\$ \subset A$ ("\$ is included in A"). "[T]he subject… is precisely constituted, which seems to be exhaustive, by any signifier insofar as he is not an element of himself", or, as he even says later, that A (or S_2) would be the "locus" where the subject appears represented or subsumed by all the other signifiers (Lacan, 1968–1969, pp. 75–76). However, \$, as A, also falls into Russell's paradox; it is neither inside nor outside {A}. As \$ is not really a signifier, but only *represented* by it, the \$ is nowhere to be definitely situated.

Thus, adding a universal quantifier, ($\forall$), we can say that $\forall_{\$}[(\$ \in A) \rightarrow (\$ \notin A)]$, which reads "for any subject, it belongs to Language if it does not belong to Language". Similarly, as a subset included in A, \$ is included-excluded, $\forall_{\$}[(\$ \subset A) \rightarrow (\$ \not\subset A)]$. For any \$, there is a belonging and an inclusion in A, while it does not belong to or is not included. This supposes an inconsistency of the set, where neither inclusion nor membership is guaranteed, that is, no possible meaning that the field of the Other may contain is guaranteed, since the Other does not seem to be outside or inside the set either.

> This demonstrates just as well, not that the subject is not included in the field of the Other, but that the point where he signifies himself as subject is exterior, in quotation marks, to the Other, that's to say, the universe of discourse.
>
> (Lacan, 1968–1969, p. 77)

The universe or domain of discourse is also a mathematical concept coming from Augustus de Morgan, but named as such by George Boole. It is a very close concept to the one W.V. Quine called, a century later, semantic holism and W. Sellar's logical space of reasons. This universe implies a set whose elements fall under the conditions of quantifiers, or, in any case, some type of formal treatment would apply to the members or included elements. The expressions used in a given language delimit a quantity or certain properties of the elements of the set.

In his *An Investigation of the Laws of Thought*, Boole (2009) characterizes the universe of discourse as a field that implicitly limits the operations of discourse, where the words and expressions used are understood by interlocutors. In his work, Boole seeks precisely to establish the laws that govern the formation of thought, deducing them through the "language of common discourse". The universe of discourse outlines the impenetrable barriers of natural language in delving to situate truth. For example, if we take the expression "men" literally, we mean *all men* that exist; we take it as universal, "all men". However, if one starts adding attributes or adjectives such as "tall men", then "tall thin men", "tall thin shy men", "tall thin shy unmarried men", etc., one can see how the elements belonging to each newly formed set diminish. The more attributes a subject, as an individual, self-assigns or has assigned to it, the more it will be excluded from that universal of "all men" and the more it will tend toward a singleton or one-point set. However, it would be a singleton flooded by the signifiers of the Other, but not turning it into one, and at the same time, increasingly excluding it from any possible universal or total inscription in the universe of discourse. Something cannot be either in or out of that universe, resists its inclusion but cannot be excluded either.

Precisely, this universe of discourse, following Kurt Gödel's theorem of incompleteness, can never be complete, *i.e.*, not everything that inhabits this universe can ever be fully proved or demonstrated, nor it is consistent, that is, contradictions and antinomies can arise at any moment, as a fact of structure. Then, in its incompleteness and inconsistency, A, place and treasure trove of signifiers and seat of discourse, will not be able to sustain everything that $ asks of it as a question or predicament, $ will only have a scope of truth to the extent that the set S_2 (knowledge) can offer to it in its limited conditions, but it will never be totalizable and consistent. The latter is summed up in another of Lacan's famous sentences: "*there is no Other of the Other*", "no metalanguage", at least not at the level of speech, in other words, there is no truth of truth.

2.2. The marge of maneuver of speech: division of the subject and the commitment

The $ is presented as divided between being subject and not being subject; it is subsumed by A and its signifiers, spoken, signified, and subjectivized by them, but also is not someone who can speak, signify, and subjectivize from them. Lacan's proposal is not structuralist, even though it draws on the linguistics of Saussure and the anthropology of Lévi-Strauss. Structuralism does not include the subject or subjectivity in its analysis of language. For the anthropologist, reality is simply the production of an unconscious reduced to structural laws where elements are logically articulated. Lacan followed this Levi-Straussian position, but he was not limited to it, that is, not only to a subject of language since he did take into account the presence of a divided subject ($) and subjectivization. So, he also thought about speech and speaking, which are not the same as language and Language (see Chapter 4). When speech is considered, there is an interlocutor, someone who receives the message. There is then an otherness at stake where there is exchange and communication. The other, as a peer, plays a role as the one we recognize and who recognizes us as valid interlocutors. This is the Hegelian movement that Lacan applies and that distances him from structuralism. Receiving your own message from another in an inverted form is what full, committed speech is based on.

Lacan identifies two types of speech: the *fides* and the feint. In *fides*, I state "You are my master" or "You are my wife"; I recognize someone first as what I am for them, and their dissent or consent determines my own status. "*You are what is still within my speech, and this I can only affirm by speaking in your place. This comes from you to find the certainty of what I pledge. This speech is speech that commits you*" (Lacan, 1955–1956, p. 37). In feint speech, I assume that the other person's speech may be intended to deceive me. Feint speech establishes and ensures a distance between subject and subject.

However, saying "you are my master" or "my wife" does not guarantee that these statements are accurate. There must be something beyond them that gives them a sense of truth and authenticity. This is the locus of the big Other, a recognized but unknown presence that is traversed by an otherness that is beyond our comprehension. It is the one who upholds the meaning of what we say and do, and it is the locus of the code that allows us to decipher and validate our speech and actions. When we utter "You are my wife" or "You are my master" to the big Other, this true and full speech establishes the place of the big absolute Other, the ultimate destination of our intentions and desires. This address commits us, even if it is false, to enter into the symbolic realm and play by its rules. "An utterance commits you to maintaining it through your discourse, or to repudiating it… to refuting it, but, even more, to complying with many things that are within the rules of the game" (Lacan, 1955–1956, p. 51).

The subject is thus caught between two structures: Language, which does not belong to the subject and to which it is alienated, and speech, in which the subject can move freely, speaking and taking the floor, which implies addressing another person. This other person may return the message in a distorted or inverted way, with contempt, misunderstanding, or aggression. However, for Lacan, speech implies agency, not structural determinism or predestination. Much of his earlier works, heavily influenced by Lévi-Strauss's reading of myths, suggest that anything happening to a subject is already laid down in some sort of empty box that was already prearranged in order for it to fill in its anticipated actions. Even if that seems to be the case for the symptom, the purpose of an analysis is to break its structural loop of deployment. It is speech and speaking that offer the chance to mobilize new subject-positions regarding one's desire and one's relation to the Other.

In any case, the speech does presuppose a big Other beyond that little other that \$ has in front of it, and that can signify and confirm the reception of the message. Perhaps the best example of how the structure of speech is disturbed is the vignette of the paranoid young woman of Seminar 3 who hallucinates her neighbor's lover insulting her when she runs up to him in the hallway of her building. She seemed to have said something as she passed, "*I've just been to the butcher's* (*charcutier*)", to which he would've responded with an insult, *Sow*! The allusion is hidden under the phrase *I've just been to the butcher's*, considering that the *charcutier*, in French, is mainly a pork meat butcher. What she was looking for was to call him a *Pig!* (Lacan, 1955–1956). If there is no Other who acknowledges receipt of the message, however, it returns to her in an inverted form and insults her; it is no longer addressed to an Other but comes back to her like a boomerang to the face.

2.3. Aphanisis *and alienation: The psychotic hallucination*

The subject ($) is an effect of the signifier, which is produced and comes from the Other. Becoming a subject takes place at the moment signification occurs, supported by the signifiers of the Other, but this event also reduces the subject to nothing more than a signifier, petrified, disappearing within the speaking process itself. For Lacan, this is the moment when the unconscious closes in on itself. Based on E. Jones, Lacan calls this moment *aphanisis*, or the fading of the subject. Enunciating signifiers condemns the speaker to being a pure effect of meaning, on the one hand, *or*, on the other, to being *aphanisis*, to vanish as being into the field of the Other. I emphasize the *or* in that phrase because that *or* is what propositional logic and set theory call a *vel*, that is, it operates as an inclusive or exclusive disjunctive for two segments of a proposition. In a proposition, a choice can be stated, that is, either it can be one object, and/or it can be the other, it does not matter which of the two (inclusive); or *else* it can only be one or the other (exclusive). Lacan, however, indicates that there is another way to define the *vel* as a more radical joining function.

> The vel of alienation is defined by a choice whose properties depend on this, that there is, in the joining, one element that, whatever the choice operating may be, has as its consequence a *neither one, nor the other*. The choice, then, is a matter of knowing whether one wishes to preserve one of the parts, the other disappearing in any case.
>
> (Lacan, 1964, p. 211)

Lacan speaks of this as the operation of *alienation* of the subject to the language of the Other. That is, whatever the choice, entering into the Language structure supposes inevitably losing something, either one of the objects of choice or both. This is the case of the assailant's famous threat, "*your money or your life?*" If one chooses the money, one loses both; if one chooses life, one loses the money. For the speaking subject, there is a similar choice between being and meaning (*sens*), where if I assume being, the meaning disappears; "it falls into non-meaning [*non-sens*]". However, if I choose meaning, only a deprived sense of the unconscious persists in the subject, and something of being is lost. The only thing in common for both choices at the point of intersection is the non-meaning where the other event that Lacan calls the operation of *separation* takes place[11]. Now, this term should be taken in its etymological sense, in Latin *se parare*, means to prepare, supply, or something produced by itself, self-engendered. This separation self-engenders as object or generates the lost object in the middle, at the point of intersection between being and meaning.

> A lack is encountered by the subject in the Other, in the very intimation that the Other makes to him by his discourse. In the intervals of the discourse of the Other, there emerges in the experience of the child something that is radically mappable, namely, *He is saying this to me, but what does he want?*

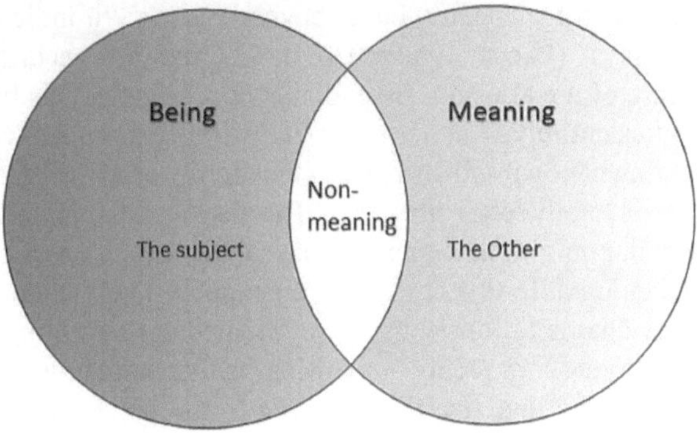

Figure 2.1

From: *The Four Fundamental Concepts of Psycho-Analysis*, 1st Edition by Jacques Lacan, © 1977 by Routledge. Reproduced by permission of Taylor & Francis Group.

> In this interval intersecting the signifiers, which forms part of the very structure of the signifier, is the locus of what… I have called metonymy. It is there that what we call desire crawls, slips, escapes, like the ferret. The desire of the Other is apprehended by the subject in that which does not work, in the lacks of the discourse of the Other, and all the child's *whys* reveal not so much an avidity for the reason of things, as a testing of the adult, a *Why are you telling me this?* ever-resuscitated from its base, which is the enigma of the adult's desire.
>
> (Lacan, 1964, p. 214)

What is the interval Lacan is speaking about? It is the result of alienation, namely, the necessary space between the couple S_1-S_2, represented here by the hyphen. The separation implies a distancing from the determination of {A} and the desire of the Other. In separation, there is a partial recuperation, through history, of the subject in fading, a self-engendering point.

Alienation is indispensable and is, as I will show in the next chapter, what occurs precisely in what Freud called the judgment of attribution. If you choose only to be, you are only an S_1, a master-signifier, but without an S_2, in that case, you are neither a subject nor can you signify. However, if you decide to include an S_2 you can no longer be solely a being, a pure presentation; you become meaning, but inescapably of the Other. So being subject $\$$ implies at any side or option to disappear, to fade behind that articulation S_1 with S_2. Thus, the arrival of S_2 results in the subject fading, disappearing, and being left divided between signifiers. In the vignette of the paranoid young woman's hallucination, she stops being in fading; she does not disappear in the hallucination as a subject, thus $S_1(\$)S_2$; what does disappear is the interval between signifiers $S_1\$S_2$, and then she is petrified by the statement from which she receives the answer. An answer that should come from the Other in the place of the interlocutor, but which happens to come from the Real of the small other which is herself. The big Other, of which I spoke above, is not beyond her partner, her interlocutor, but is beyond herself; "it indicates itself in a beyond of what it says" (Lacan, 1955–1956, p. 52), and this, according to Lacan, is the very structure of the allusion. He explains how, in psychotic hallucinations, the subject identifies entirely with her ego, with whom she speaks while speaking about herself, finding her own self stripped of the dignity of a true speaker. The *I*, as a linguistic shifter, is totally left in abeyance. The absence of *aphanisis* and interval is the key to understanding what happens in psychotic decompensation (delusional states and hallucinations). In this case, one can suppose that the statement of this young woman was unable to follow its intention "without detaching itself from it by the dash that introduces the reply—opposing its disparaging antistrophe to the grumbling of the strophe that was thus restored to the patient with the index of the I…" (Lacan, 1959, pp. 448–449). This suggests that in psychotic hallucination there is no Other who issues a response, or a reply coming from elsewhere, that is, from another intention that could respond to it differently in an antistrophe. Statement and reply are grounded in and emerge from the same place.

The $ is presented as divided, between being subjected and not being subjected to {A}; it does not seem to be able to configure itself as someone who is within the set or outside it, subsumed by {A} and its signifiers or not really. The divided subject is divided, precisely because it is caught in an in-between, sometimes aware and in control of its utterances and intentions, others totally submerged by it, or felt excluded from the chain. So, it is spoken, signified, and subjectivized by {A}, while unable to *totally and freely* speak, signify, and subjectivize even if belonging to it. So, how does $ *differ* from the S_2 that embodies that Other *without completely dissociating* itself from it? Another way of formulating the previous question is: How is the $, as a subject of speech (*parole*), not completely trapped, fused with the signifiers and signifieds of {A}, while not being radically separated from them either?

Note

1 Lacan refers later in Seminar 11 to separation as "the weak point of the primal dyad of the signifying articulation… It is in the interval between these two signifiers [S_1-S_2] that resides the desire offered to the mapping of the subject in the experience of the discourse of the Other, of the first he has to deal with… the mother" (Lacan, 1964, p. 218). The mother's desire will remain enigmatic and confusing to the child; it is in this lack that the child subject is constituted as such: the lack is instantiated by the child's *aphanisis*.

3

Negation and name

Founders of the subject

3.1. The judgments of attribution and existence: the emergence of the Real

The answers to the questions with which the previous chapter closed come from two proposals: the negation in the judgments of attribution and existence, and the proper name of the void. Negation and being named (and later naming) come as potentialities for the uses of language and the process of subjectivization. This means that the subject counts as multiple-one, but without being co-opted by the signifiers of the Other.

In the case of judgments of attribution and existence, both imply a form of constitutive negation (*Verneinung*). According to Lacan, Freud was the first person to suggest a form of entry into the judicative world of being, starting from a judgment of attribution linked to the oral drive: "*I like this, thus I shall take it and put it inside of me*" or "*this is disagreeable, thus it shall remain outside of me*". The toddler, of course, does not enunciate them as strict propositions; thus, their enabling resides as mere pre-predicative judgments in the form of negation/affirmation, expulsion/incorporation. Lacan considers that the first form of expulsion (negation) of the conditions of the object precedes its imaginary re-presentation (*Darstellung*). This judgment of attribution (as the first form of expulsion of the object and its attributes) is the "primordial condition for something from the [R]eal to come to offer itself up to the revelation of being [...] since it is only afterwards that anything whatever can be found there as existent [*comme étant*]" (Lacan, 1954, p. 323). In addition, this type of judgment establishes a sort of first adumbration to the later use of signifiers; a dialectic of incorporation/expulsion, affirmation/negation, pleasure/unpleasure, when everything appears at first to the toddler as identical to themselves, as part of themselves. The introduction of expulsion, the original repression (*Urverdrängung*), "without which the operation of introjection would have no meaning" (Hyppolite, 1954, p. 751), implies a first step towards the world of Language.

DOI: 10.4324/9781032663616-5

This original repression supposes the expulsion of something from that primordial object towards a "locus", which is actually the subject's own history (something mythical, as Hyppolite points out), "a place where he can grab hold of it" (Lacan, 1954, p. 324), to narrate something about itself; it is the necessary articulation between the Symbolic and the Imaginary, allowing a glimpse of the Real. In this, reality accommodates itself as a result of the knotting of the Symbolic and the Imaginary, enabling us to identify the presence of what was already there:

> the [R]eal—as that which is excised [*verworfen*] from the primordial symbolization. [...] the subject can see emerge something of it in the form of a thing [*Ding*], which is far from being an object that satisfies him and which involves its present intentionality...
>
> (Lacan, 1954, pp. 324–325)

Based on Freud's case of the Wolf-Man, Lacan interprets Sergei Pankejeff's childhood hallucination of accidentally excising his pinkie with a knife, and feeling a great deal of anxiety, as

> the Imaginary echo, which arises as a response to a point of reality that belongs to the limit where it has been excised [*verworfen*] from the Symbolic. This means that the sense that something is unreal is exactly the same phenomenon as the sense of reality...
>
> (Lacan, 1954, p. 326)

Pankejeff's experience turns into a mirage when the void of the Thing is revealed as Real before this subjective fading, it becomes clear that the amputation of his finger does not exist, does not correspond, and does not match any judgment of existence. Anxiety appears before the evidence of the Thing as void of meaning and impossible, as the encounter with the Real, that which is cut off from the Symbolic and the Imaginary.

It is here, in his *Response to Jean Hyppolite's commentary on Freud's 'Verneinung'*, that for the first time, Lacan uses the concept of *Verwerfung*, translating it as excision (*retranchement*). It is clearly not the same as repression, since in this excision, an element is expelled from the Symbolic, while in repression, the eviction occurs within Symbolic memory. By 1954, *Verwerfung* had figured as a fundamental step in the formation of reality, as that which opposes the *Bejahung* (affirmation) in the judgment of attribution, the primary experience of that which is definitively expelled from the Symbolic towards the Real. "*Verwerfung* thus cuts short any manifestation of the Symbolic order" (Lacan, 1954, p. 323), and if any signifier or presentation did not pass through the Symbolic, they would appear in the Real in the form of a hallucination or a delusion. I will show in Chapter 5 how this concept will be applied to foreclosure.

It could be inferred that immediately after judgments of attribution arise existence judgments of the type: "*This is not my dream... or my representation, but an object*" (Lacan, 1955–1956, p. 150) (again, the toddler is yet incapable of forming explicit propositions of this kind, but it can pre-predicatively acknowledge them). This type of judgment entails both the first-person apprehension of the presentation of the object and a second form of negation that already implies a reality-testing and a reality-ego, or, at least, what we could simply call a judgment by correspondence. *Reality* would be the presentation to the senses of the object and its correspondence to the state of affairs in the world. The negation of what is perceived when it does not correspond to the state of affairs would be a first form of apprehension of a shared objective reality. However, this judgment, Freud reminds us, would necessarily entail for the toddler the presence of a "fellow-human being" (usually one that embodies a first satisfaction/hostile object) that would assent or dissent upon the judgment. It is through the intermediary of the Other (both as a fellow being and source of reference of the judgment) that the subject cognizes (Freud, 1895, p. 331).

3.2. Negation as reality constitution

Memory, together with the apprehension of reality, depends on the fact of remembering and re-presenting (*darstellen*) an absent object, even an already lost object, that brought the first forms of satisfaction and pleasure to the body from the Other. Negation (*Versagung*), which Strachey translates as "failure" in Freud's "Letter 52 to Fliess" (though it is sometimes translated as "frustration" by others), is what opens the way to the first form of repression in the toddler, but more importantly, a first form of putting perceptions into signs, allowing the implementation of the linguistic-affective memory (Freud, 1896, p. 235; Lacan, 1955–1956, p. 156). Lacan interprets this letter to Fliess as a description of the minimum adumbration necessary for Language to enable memory and historicization. By negating some of the fantasized attributes of the object, the original repression (*Urverdrängung*) takes place, where the subject ascribes existence *not solely* by perceiving the object as a state of affairs, but as it tries to find it once again in its fantasized-longed-for[1] features. This is negation, which institutes and finds a "not belonging to" property of the legality of sets ($\alpha \notin \beta$) while negating the legality of this property through the frame of fantasy (($\$ \lozenge a) \rightarrow \neg \alpha \notin \beta$).

So, both types of judgment, attribution and existence, can clearly be sought as pre-predicative, that is, a set of multiples that count-as-one qua an "object", but which affect us in the background as already present to consciousness in an "objective apprehension", the perception of the object having its own horizon (Husserl, 1973, § 8). *But Husserl's objective apprehension falls short*; this is the teaching of Freud, because the subject seeks to find again the satisfaction of the object of illusion, so the aim of reality-testing is "to find an object in real perception, which corresponds to the one presented, but to refind such an object, to convince oneself that it is still there. [...] The reproduction of a perception as presentation is not always a faithful one" (Freud, 1925, pp. 237–238). Reality-testing and the pleasure principle will always be in tension in any perception when a judgment of predication is performed. Objective presentation and re-presentation are never guaranteed according to Freud, their objectivity is imbued with the pleasure principle's tendencies.

Therefore, the judgment of existence is not only pre-predicative because of what the outside traces or structures as a figure-ground, as a horizon of meaning, but also because from the inside out, that which is introjected counts as an attribute of the "reality" of the re-presented object. Symbolic negation facilitates the divorce between the subjective (the inside) and the objective (outside, or the field of objects) and is key to opening the way to this dialectic, to this possibility of not being prey to the field of objects or submerged by the signifiers of the Other. It makes it easier to cope with the tension between the pleasure and the reality principles, maintaining a sort of balance. The presentation of objects does not correspond with the maintenance of pleasure, or at least, the re-presentation is inveigled with pleasure principle tendencies, which may disregard any correspondence with the world's state of affairs. The objective presentation and re-presentation of objects are always permeated and distorted by this inherent tension.

3.3. To name as entry into existence and the count

What remains of the relationship between *perceptum* and re-presentation (*Darstellung*) apprehension once a judgment is made? This time, however, I am talking about a predicative judgment, that is, when the multiple begins to count-as-one, $p \rightarrow x$, if *p*resented then x, that x configuring an appearance of statable oneness, its status of membership in a set by predicating the presentation. In this case, Badiou's ontological position assumes that between the presentation of the object as structure and the presentation of the object as a structur*ed*-presentation, or between the presented consistency and the inconsistency of what-will-have-been-presented, *there is nothing*. The Real is the only thing that limits the effect of the count. "The 'nothing' is what names the unperceivable gap...", "names the undecidable of presentation which is its unpresentable", or is a "phantom of inconsistency" (Badiou, 2005, pp. 54–55). Just as for there to be a multiple that counts as one, lending itself to a structured presentation or under which an object falls, *first* there must be something that aims to count-as-one (a multiple of multiples) but under which no object falls. That is, nought and the empty set {ø}, *i.e.*, the only thing that can come to Language as a multiple of "nothing", as a non-appearance of presentation. The empty set is non-extensional, that is, it cannot be replaced by anything other than itself; it only finds equivalence in its own inexistence.

For a multiple to begin to be counted as a consistent one, like several-ones counted by the action of the structure, one must first be able to name it. Only named, it ceases to be the unpresentable, the void. It begins to count-as-one in

Language when $\{ø\}$ (empty set) receives its name, the name-of-the-empty, since the only element that will constitute it will be its own name; only its denomination belongs to it, $ø \in \{ø\}$. According to Badiou, the name fulfills the function of a "suture-to-being", a suture that allows the multiplicity to be contained as the noun-phrase of any proposition. This generates the idea of oneness, but this idea is only an apparent assumption.

> I can thus consider that the set $\{ø\}$, which counts-as-one the result of the originary count—the one-multiple which is the name of the void—is the forming-into-one [*mise-en-un*] of this name. Therein the one acquires no further being than that conferred upon it operationally by being the structural seal of the multiple.
>
> (Badiou, 2005, p. 91)

Being able *to name* the void, what is not presented, favors the idea of an apparent oneness and suggests that $\{ø\}$ is the first singleton of the forming-into-one of any multiple; it is the first unpresentable presence of the Thing. Here we can ask ourselves: How do we go from the Thing, unpresentable and unnamable, to the signifier, presented and namable? "A situation never proposes anything other than multiples woven from ones, and the law of laws is that nothing limits the effect of the count" (Badiou, 2005, p. 54). This means that the count cannot be stopped; the multiple will become one as an imperative logical necessity. As a one, that which will seal or amalgamate the multiple will be the name that is attributed to it; it will become a set under a designation, existent. We are subjects to a large extent because the proper name comes to cover, not a great particularity, but a crack, the constitutive lack (see Chapter 5), and the Thing that opens to the void. Lacan alludes that the proper name serves to stitch together with a degree of consistency the inconsistent being of the multiplicity conforming the subject (Lacan, 1964–1965, April 7th, 1965).

3.4. The name and species as a logical operator: introducing meaning

However, the proper name has a drawback, which Claude Lévi-Strauss briefly explores in his book *La pensée sauvage*: Does the proper name designate a set or is it a singleton, *i.e.*, does the name belong as the only element of the set? In other words, does the proper name make its bearer count as one, as one of the particular (which is articulated with the universal), that is, as one who belongs to a class by its surname ("as a result of their practically unlimited extension and their fundamental undifferentiation") or is individual and particular because of its name, who is "named only because [it] could not be signified (Gardiner)" (Lévi-Strauss, 2021, p. 194)? Here lies the problem of the universal and the particular.

According to Lévi-Strauss, thought intrinsically seeks a coherent organization, classification, and articulation of the world's data. In this sense, the classification, however arbitrary and heterogeneous it may be, "preserves the wealth and diversity of the inventory. In deciding that everything must be accounted for, it facilitates the constitution of a 'memory'" (Lévi-Strauss, 2021, p. 19). The opposition of minimal forms of presentation, related by contiguity or similarity, is the structure of Language. These oppositions occur through the possibility of attributing signifiers to them, that is, sets of phonemes and semanthemes, which make this antagonism *ex*-ist, favoring the classification of presentations. Being able to name, as a proper or common name, seems to configure the field of fundamental oppositions, splits, and successive superimpositions that facilitate the creation of a concept (Lacan, 1964–1965).

In this logic, the totem, the surname, the gender, etc., according to Lévi-Strauss, contributed to ethnology and linguistics with the notion of *species* as a logical operator. This operator makes it possible to index apparently distant fields and sets at the classificatory level. It achieves this by widening the limits of the initial set of species, favoring universalization, or by expanding the classificatory attributes of the natural limits to particularize; that is, it props up individualities (Lévi-Strauss, 2021, p. 185). In this same vein, the concept of NotF is a relevant organizer, close to the species-as-operator, that seeks to link that impossible extrapolation of the particular with the universal through the mediation of the idea of a set. The symbol that is the species-as-operator is an invention of the Symbolic that allows us to solve, through writing, an entire problem of the limitations of the Imaginary and the Symbolic.

In Boolean algebra, a logical connective or operator consists of a term facilitating the connection of two sentences while maintaining grammatical coherence, creating a compound sentence. However, it seems that it is more accurate to focus on the use of the notion of species, which Lévi-Strauss draws from A. Comte and his *Cours de philosophie positive*. In Lesson 52 he talks about what he believes is the basis of the transition from fetishistic (animism) to polytheistic societies (Lévi-Strauss, 2021; Comte, 2000). The concept of species would be a step towards inductive and observational thinking, when, in a culture, a single object is attributed with the properties of a fetish, containing an individual and concrete nature, power or magic. However, the prolonged observation of the object and the suppositions that were attributed to it may be modified or abandoned. This usually means the advent of deities as abstract figures capable of a certain power or condition, who exercise dominance over many bodies with certain characteristics, while the fetish only does so over the one in which it resides.

> Thus when the oaks of a forest, in their likeness to each other, suggested certain general phenomena, the abstract being in whom so many fetiches coalesced was no fetich, but the god of the forest. Thus, the intellectual transition from fetichism to polytheism is neither more nor less than the ascendancy of specific over individual ideas... Polytheism itself might have been primitive in certain cases, where the individual had a strong natural tendency to abstraction, while his contemporaries, being more impressible than reasonable, were more struck by differences than by resemblances.
>
> (Comte, 2000, p. 26)

Comte supposes here the birth of inductive thinking as the arrival of the idea of condensing under a name a certain degree of common properties among a diversity of bodies, thus generating the term species as a logical operator. The proper name counts both as part of a class and a social bond, as well as the designation of a unique and unrepeatable subject. It moves from an individual conception to a specific one and vice-versa. The signifier NotF comes into operation as a naming function, as a metaphor (the Paternal metaphor), which names not the Father but the subject that bears the name given by the naming function. The metaphor is the replacement of a signifier for another signifier maintaining signification. This implies departing from the void that is the Thing when naming objects or naming multiples that count-as-one, by attributing a signifier to any event. To name is to metaphorize, it is replacing an event for what can designate it, the eventful site on the edge of the void for a name (see Chapter 11). Hence the famous phrase by Lacan: "The symbol first manifests itself as the killing of the *thing*, and this death results in the endless perpetuation of the subject's desire" (Lacan, 1953a, p. 262). The signifier NotF would offer the introduction of the symbol and the chain of signifiers in the speaking human subject that articulates them to the field of demand (requests) and desire. When the child says that the dog goes woof-woof and the cat meow-meow, it disconnects the cry from the referent and "raises the sign to the function of signifier, and reality to the sophistics of signification" (Lacan, 1960, p. 682). The price to pay, however, is the "death" (masking) of the Thing and the loss of the object. However, this same operator safeguards the subject from the return of the object in its Real form; as long as it sustains the framework of the fundamental fantasy the object will be kept away as a pure semblance, a veil (I'll address this further in Chapter 12).

This logical operator also includes the possibility of placing boundaries between sets, of becoming a member or a subset, or of not doing so; of holding oneness or multiplicity; of maintaining delimited borders of space-time—not only of the One, the multiple, and the nought—by the knotting of the Symbolic, the Real, and the Imaginary around the gap. However, for this to happen, as I'll try to demonstrate in Chapter 5, the extraction of object *a* must have occurred. Language involves more than just distinguishing between signifiers or engaging in a play of oppositions. As G. Morel emphasizes, it also entails the isolation and singular essence of a signifier, in its self-referentiality. This is a concept Lacan coined as the unary trait (*trait unaire*). It represents that which simultaneously sets distinctions while remaining singular and incomparable, identical to itself yet distinct to the others, akin to one (or the amount of the set "identical with 0"). This notion serves as the genesis of the count, akin to the notches etched by a prehistoric hunter onto the ribs of an Ice Age mammal. It might sound strange to think of difference as something connected to oneness, but that is the key to how we understand the world. When we seek to distinguish between two entities, to compare or contrast them, we assign each with a particular trait or characteristic, essentially an attribute, and then discern differences among these attributes. This "identification-differentiation-classification" process is the foundation of traditional logic systems like Aristotle's *Categories*, where things are grouped based on shared attributes. It's like a language game with two sides: the order of the signifier with its opposites (think day versus night), and the way we build propositions (subject-copula-attribute) (Morel, 2011).

Note

1 It must be specified here that studies carried out in the 1970s and 1980s indicated that representational thought appears in infants between 9 and 24 months of age (Stern, 1998; Cavell, 1996). This could open several possibilities in interpreting what Freud proposes, or either the original repression occurs after the ninth month or, approximately, the first year, or when the infant fully enters language, before weaning. Or it enters the logic of the Freudian *proton pseudos* (Freud, 1895), where the symptom occurs in two logical times, that is, retroaction (*Nachträglichkeit*) generates *post hoc* effects. Satisfaction arises only after the fact as an experience lived from the memory or the assumption of memory.

4

Language, the zero-value signifier, and the signifier of the lack in the Other, S(Ⱥ)

4.1. The metastructure of presentation and of language {A}

Ferdinand de Saussure, considered one of the great revolutionaries of linguistics, proposed making a distinction between acts of speech (*langage*), language (*langue*), and speaking (*parole*). The language (*langue*) is a social product of the faculty of Language (W. Baskin translates *langage* as "acts of speech", but I will employ the word Language, with a capital L), together with the conventions adopted by a social group to exercise that power (Saussure, 2011, p. 9). "Language [*langue*] is speech [*langage*] less speaking [*parole*]. It is the whole set of linguistic habits that allow an individual to understand and be understood" (Saussure, 2011, p. 77). However, the translation into English of these three terms is quite complex, and one generally only seeks to make the contrast between the language (*langue*) and the speaking (*parole*), neglecting the Language (*langage*). The latter is a more encompassing set of articulated laws under which a diversity of subsets is included but not necessarily united, intersected, or even closely identical. The elements of each subset are heterogeneous among themselves but obey the same laws and metastructure of the Language set. Thus, one can speak of a Language (*langage*) of informatics, of signs (for the hearing impaired), nonverbal, myth, etc.

Saussure continues his linguistic theorizing by pointing out that for there to be a language (*langue*), there must be a community of speakers; therefore, it would not exist without the social interaction. The language is constituted by the linguistic sign, which forms a unit comprised of a concept and a sound-image (or acoustic image); but that sound-image is not the mere sound and the enunciated phonemes but rather "the psychological imprint of the sound, the impression it makes on our senses" (Saussure, 2011, p. 66). Saussure prefers to call the concept the signified, the sound-image the signifier, and this whole set the sign. Both one and the other participate in a system of oppositions within a grammar or syntax (Saussure, 2011, p. 66).

What do the laws of language consist of? The set $\{ø, \{S_1\}, \{S_2\}\}$ that we saw in Chapter 2 would appear as the minimal metastructure of {A}. However, without {A} being equivalent with $\{ø, \{S_1\}, \{S_2\}\}$, the former is an essentially different multiple from the latter; there is extensionality but no equivalence. The latter is

DOI: 10.4324/9781032663616-6

more "a metastructure, another count, which 'completes' the first in that it gathers together all the sub-compositions of internal multiples, all the inclusions" (Badiou, 2005, p. 83). For the constitutive void—pure chaos—to not appear in a presentation, something must escape its count; the structure of {A} must enjoy a metastructure, *i.e.*, a structure of the structure, without this implying an *ad infinitum* regression. "The consistency of presentation thus requires that all structure be doubled by a metastructure [that] secures the former against any fixation of the void" (Badiou, 2005, pp. 93–94). Badiou deduces the metastructure from what he calls the theorem of the *point of excess*, which itself comes from the Zermelo–Fraenkel power-set axiom. A power-set is the "grand" set that contains all possible subsets of an original set. In other words, an initial set, together with all the subsets that compose it, can be reduced to a one, to a single power-set, codified as P(A). This P(A) would be the largest babushka doll containing the smaller ones, A, $\{S_1\}$, $\{S_1, S_2\}$, etc. Badiou's proposal is that in that P(A) there is a multiple that does not belong to the initial set; he calls this multiple the point of excess.

Before we move on, however, let's keep in mind something that was said from the beginning about set theory: *being included* ($\subset$) *is not the same as belonging or being a member* ($\in$) of a set. The power-set P(A) of all the subsets of the *now* subset A is essentially different from A itself, it poses a second count, necessarily. Then we have that $A \subset P(A)$ but not that $A \in P(A)$. If the latter were the case, it would be Russell's paradox (see Chapter 2). If we start from the principle that $A \notin A$ and we assume that the subset $A \in P(A)$, we realize that this subset is no other than A itself, then necessarily $A \in A$, thus falling into a contradiction. "This is to say, *no multiple is capable of forming-a-one out of everything it includes.* [...] Inclusion is in irremediable excess of belonging" (Badiou, 2005, p. 85).

The metastructure is a point of excess, something that constitutes and shapes the presentation but that is not namable, this is, it is inexistent, it functions as an unnamable container but cannot be a member of itself. To a certain extent, Lacan hints at this power-set, when in *On a question prior to any possible treatment of psychosis* he admits the existence of an Other of the Other, especially with this somewhat complex but categorical sentence at the end of the text:

> This is the term in which the process by which the signifier was "unleashed" in the [R]eal culminates, after the Name-of-the-Father began to collapse—the latter being the signifier which, in the Other, qua locus of the signifier, is the signifier of the Other qua locus of the law.
>
> (Lacan, 1959, p. 485)

This indicates that for Lacan there would be two Others, one who is the Other of the signifier, and the Other of the law. There would be a large set containing itself: a signifier of the Other. The Other is a set that contains itself as a subset, and, furthermore, is included at the same time in that of the law. Lacan seems to take NotF as a specific signifier with a single function, operating as the Other of the Other. That is, we can say that the NotF signifier is sustained as a metastructure, or the power-set.

This is close to Lacan's definition of what a structure is: "a group of elements forming a covariant set" where the "structure is always established by referring something coherent to something else, which is complementary to it" (Lacan, 1955–1956, p. 183). For Lacan, the psychic structure presupposes the signifier. Thus, to be interested in the structure is to be interested in the signifier and the properties of the Other, {A}. The term "covariant set" is important here because it means that the signifier on its own would be worthless. It needs interrelationships with other signifiers to acquire a position in the set. What would then be the metastructure of a structure, and what redoubles it by turning it into P(A)? Badiou replies that it would only be a "part" of the situation, "being neither points nor the whole". A part is a sub-multiple, a multiple made up of multiple-ones. Now, Badiou emphasizes that a consistent multiplicity, counted-as-one, belongs to a situation, and that the subset of these multiplicities is included in the situation. However, only that which belongs to the situation *shows up* in the presentation. Only that which belongs is presented, that which is included is assumed. This is where the metastructure comes to play a role. In this case, the metastructure of {A}, of Language, is a signifier that is included but does not belong to the set, or in any case, it's the irreducible form of the signifier, a consistent multiple. The NotF would be the name of the metastructure of the signifier, not insofar as it is a Saussurian sign or a signified tied to a signifier. Here I return to the key role played by the first judgment of existence; this judgment supposes a metastructure given by a "primordial process", a process "of exclusion of an original within, which is not of a bodily within but that of an initial body of signifiers. It's inside this primordial body that Freud posits the constitution of a world of reality..." (Lacan, 1955–1956, p. 150). It is not something corporeal that is excluded towards the outside, but a first body of the signifier, a first minimal, irreducible form of it. Form in which the entire {A} will immediately depart together with its elements and subsets and which will become a compositional part of the subject's speech and use of language. The NotF is that first body or form of signifier that, in psychosis, for Lacan, finds itself rejected or—to use the term he uses for the first time in *On a question prior...*—foreclosed (*verworfen*). Now, this does not mean that the psychotic subject is therefore prey to absolute chaos in its use of language (*langue*) and cannot really access it, even though that may be the case (*e.g.*, severe schizophrenia in childhood or profound autism). However, the foreclosure of this signifier will make it difficult for the psychotic to enter the world of discourse since this primordial form is key "in the organization of language in order for memory and historicization to work", considering this body of signifier will serve nothing if it does not come into operation in the history of the subject, especially in its sexual desire and jouissance, level at which the law is introduced for the first time (Lacan, 1955–1956, p. 156).

4.2. The zero symbolic value of the first body of signifier

These operations of opposition between signs, Lévi-Strauss reminds us, can be seen in all kinds of spoken or natural languages when one signifier can signify two antithetical operations (Lévi-Strauss, 1987). Following Marcel Mauss and his analysis of the term "mana", he points out that there would be certain signifiers that would be "floating" and bearing a *zero symbolic value* since they are not directly opposed to any other signifier. Terms like "mana", "wakan", and "orenda", or simply their usage, ritualized practices such as the "north-south axis" for the Bororo of Brazil (Lévi-Strauss, 1963), employed by various indigenous peoples, "can [have] any value at all, provided it is still part of the available reserve and is not already, as the phonologist says, a term in a set" (Lévi-Strauss, 1987, p. 64; Zafiropoulos, 2010). A similar use is made of the terms *machin* or *truc*, in French, or *vaina*, in Spanish, which turn out to be floating signifiers even if they have their own "univocal" signified. Then, the floating signifier, as a signifying body, must be available as a subset of {A} but cannot *yet* be an element of the set. The *yet* is important because it implies a between-two, precisely because of its floating character. It has to be inside, but at the same time outside, under the condition of being ready to enter again. The floating signifier favors the possibility of maneuvering with language since it offers a body. It configures the assumption of positions when we use speech (and more structurally, discourse), that is, by allowing the issuance of diverse propositional statements, reducing terms, filling them with meaning, playing with language while we are agents endowed with a degree of freedom in its use, etc. The signifier NotF would become a floating signifier, which is why Lacan suggested in the failed Seminar that he could not carry out entirely in 1963, titled *On the Names-of-the-Father* (Lacan, 1963), that it could be pluralized.

Now, this proposal of the NotF as a signifier of zero value is suggested by M. Zafiropoulos (2010). The same symbolic value would be represented by myth and its structure.

> Myth itself could, as a consequence, play the role of these exceptional signifiers that permit thought to operate. We have placed Lacan's 'invention' of the Name-of-Father in the class of terms that have a zero symbolic value… To follow Lévi-Strauss, we could say that the stability of myth, which is indicated by the ease with which it can be translated, is in proximity with the proper name, which ensures the durability of identification in the set of all possible worlds.
>
> (Zafiropoulos, 2010, pp. 173–174)

The myth can figure as a NotF, a series of signifiers articulated within a minimal structure, or metastructure, which is sustained by a designation (a name) following the pattern of the myth formula proposed by Lévi-Strauss (Lévi-Strauss, 1963, p. 228). I will not go right now into detail about this formula (see Chapter 10). However, I seek to indicate, as I will do in more detail in Part 2, that the NotF does not allow any kind of concept or specific signification; its "floating" character implies that various instituted signifiers are associated with it and around a specific function, that of legislating and instituting. Lacan always emphasized that the NotF is the promoter of the Law (Lacan, 1959, p. 482). For him, this means that "the law of man has been the law of [L]anguage" (Lacan, 1953a, p. 225), and "is in the *name of the father* that we must recognize the basis of the symbolic function which, since the dawn of historical time, has identified his person with the figure of the law" (Lacan, 1953a, p. 230).

But is the law the Other of the Other, of {A}? Is there the truth of truth? Almost simultaneously with the declaration of NotF as an "Other of the Other", in the Seminar, *Desire and Its Interpretation*—carried out practically in parallel with the publication of *On a question prior...*—Lacan will affirm in his interpretation of Hamlet's actions that "there is no Other of the Other" (Lacan, 1958–1959, p. 298), that is, the NotF is not a guarantee of anything, since the subject has to confront the incompleteness and inconsistency of A, that is, the signifier of the lack.

4.3. Is lack signifying? The signifier of the lack in the Other

Despite this idea of zero symbolic value and its assemblage within a metastructure that legalizes a set, provoking a "universe of discourse", Lacan will propose something that does not allow reducing "mana" to a lack or a S_1 but to something that seems even more paradoxical as a signifier. In those zero-valued terms, there is already a signifier with a use, which belongs to the signifier's set, $\{S_1\}$. An eventful lack must be written by means of a signifier that does not seem to count in {A} but that counts in it at the same time. The loss of the object installing the lack is constitutive, as I will show in the following chapter. How should one signify the lack without counting it as an element employed in ordinary language, that is, that it can be written? The moment we name a lack and use it as a designator, lack disappears. So, Lacan proposes S(Ⱥ) (capital S stands for signifier, A with a bar is the lack in the Other), thus the "signifier of a lack in the Other, a lack inherent in the Other's very function as treasure trove of signifiers" (Lacan, 1960, p. 693). However, using S(Ⱥ) does not fill the lack because it is a rigid designator; it does not contradict itself when writing the lack because Lacan supposes it to be logically extensional to $\sqrt{-1}$. He continues with his dissertation, affirming that

> Claude Levi-Strauss, commenting on Mauss' work, no doubt wished to see in mana the effect of a zero symbol. But it seems that what we are dealing with in our case is rather the signifier of the lack of this zero symbol. This is why, at the risk of incurring a certain amount of opprobrium, I have indicated how far I have gone in distorting mathematical algorithms in my own use of them: for example, my use of the symbol, $\sqrt{-1}$, also written *i* in the theory of complex numbers, can obviously be justified only if I give up any claim to its being able to be used automatically in subsequent operations.
>
> (Lacan, 1960, pp. 695–696)

This signifier of the lack is of the lack, but without being able to be counted in any set, unless, that is, the set of imaginary numbers. It is an unpronounceable signifier, but it operates whenever a proper name is used or pronounced. Why is that S(Ⱥ) like the square root of -1? Because $\sqrt{-1}$ does not inhabit the set of real numbers, it is an imaginary number to which one can try to calculate its value, but one can never coalesce the calculation into a real number or a signifier; one will only be able to name it as such, as √-1 or *i*. It is paradoxical because this peculiar signifier is what inscribes what is not there—a structural lack. This signifier of the lack is precisely the fact that the analysand, in their analysis, reaches the point of impasse in which there is no metadiscourse, no truth of the truth, and where this Other shows incomplete and inconsistent. They finally run into the emptiness that does *not* embody this signifier. The point is to realize that they are castrated, that they do not possess what would come to complete that Other, nor that this Other has what the analysand would need to be completed and consistent. This S(Ⱥ) is the central question that Lacan situates in the place of "what am I?" A space that seems to remain unanswered, opening towards a lack. However, it is a valid and necessary lack for the subject to assume a subjectivity, a place in the world as a subject who commits and lives its own desire. This signifier is the place where that which this author designates with the highly complex concept of jouissance resides, "whose absence would render the universe vain" (Lacan, 1960, p. 694). The following chapter offers the perspective of two foundational moments in all speaking beings that imply original repression and castration.

5

Castration and the "extraction of object *a*", the offshoots of the Oedipus complex

> Socio-cultural symbolism effects an identical registration of self on the part of the subject. For example, when the child takes his place in the family constellation on an equal footing with a forename and a surname as well as the third party position he occupies with regard to the parental couple, he recuperates himself as a distinct entity as opposed to the primary merging of himself with his mother. For the Lacanians, access to socio-cultural symbolism, to a socialized existence, is realized by going beyond the Oedipal drama. [...]
>
> If symbolism is then a human dimension or even a positive human condition in that it socializes and organizes man, it also presents the disadvantage of formalizing the vital individual experience. What is more, symbolization is human, it is the work of human minds, which implies from the start: imperfection, reduction, arbitrariness, submission to external constraints and a partial failure to recognize its own mechanisms. The impossible task of symbolization in the broadest sense of the word is to organize at its own level the multiplicity of 'vital human conditions.' Each type of social organization has only been able to respond to these necessities in a partial way, accentuating certain aspects of life at the expense of others and therefore effecting repression.
>
> Thus, for example, our occidental, patriarchal societies have given what is universal in the Oedipal drama a particular dramatized form which leads to the male and female types of castration complexes with which we are acquainted.
>
> (Lemaire, 1977, pp. 57–58)
>
>

5.1. Child psychosis: an empirical approach to the intersubjective and relational ground of psychosis

This long epigraph of Anika Lemaire's work, published during Lacan's lifetime, indicates the effects of symbolization and the entry into the symbolic world of human culture. Castration appears as required to enter the circuit of the universe of discourse; it is another way of establishing a loss, or a second type of loss. Based on Freud and the Oedipus complex, the S(Ⱥ) is a second type of lack instituted by the

DOI: 10.4324/9781032663616-7

action of castration, or it could also be read as "extraction of object *a*" (Londoño, Gil, and Marín, 2023; Lacan, 1959, p. 487).

The psychoanalytic work with psychotic children, such as the case of Melanie Klein's *Dick* or Rosine Lefort's *Robert* (Lacan, 1953–1954, lectures VII and VIII), were inspirational for Lacan's theoretical proposal on the relational bases of psychosis and the Oedipus complex. If a social ontology of psychosis can be posited, it is precisely in the intersubjective game in which Lacan locates it in his first seminars. The Oedipus and castration complexes exemplify how language, knowledge, desire, and jouissance are established or absent, delineating a subject's psychic structure. In Lacanian psychoanalysis, a subject's actions and psychic structure make sense a posteriori (*nachträglich*), based on their biography and early interpersonal relationships regarding knowledge, jouissance, and the object *a* (desire) (Lacan, 1968–1969, pp. 331–332). *How did the immediate social agents in a microsystem, or caregivers, offer knowledge about jouissance and desire to a subject? What social fact at stake as a causal process within this social ontology is relevant in the formation of psychosis?*

I take here the writings of a contemporary psychoanalyst of Lacan who worked with children at the New York State Psychiatric Institute and had the opportunity to see first-hand cases of infantile psychosis, a topic to which Margaret Mahler contributed for many years. If anything characterizes psychoses in children, it is a deficiency in the symbolization and configuration of the body image and body experience, all mediated by the Other. For example, what she cataloged as "symbiotic psychoses" are paradigmatic and coincide to a certain point with the causal explanation that Lacan seeks to outline about psychosis in Seminars 3, 4, and 5, and *On a question prior to any possible treatment of psychosis* (Lacan, 1959).

Mahler described in the early 1950s this type of psychosis occurring in young children who failed to go through the phase of separation-individuation in relation to the maternal object and remained hampered in a symbiotic phase. This author portrayed various types of behavior and attitudes on the part of the mother that could cause or worsen prepsychotic stages or transient symbiotic psychoses. For instance, the "well-known parasitic, infantilizing mother who needs to continue her overprotection beyond the stage when it's beneficial. This attitude becomes an engulfing threat, detrimental to the child's normal disengagement and individuation…" (Mahler and Gosliner, 1955, p. 201). For Mahler, there would be in these "symbiotic" children a fusion of the self and the non-self, making it impossible for them to emotionally distinguish what they are experiencing from what the mother is experiencing. The fact of being separated from their mother would generate an anxiety that is sometimes self-injurious and aggressive, all in order to preserve the "unconditionally omnipotent symbiotic unity". In this symbiotic phase with the predominance of a feeling of union with the maternal object as a partial object, the source of her tensions is internal and what calms them both comes from outside; another object exerts some presence or act that facilitates this appeasement. This leads to a "rudimentary ego differentiation" during the first year of life. The infant begins to separate itself and its mental representations from the mother's. Mahler indicates how certain environments are not favorable, due to the presence of traumatic situations within them, for individuation and disengagement in the formation of an ego autonomy (Mahler, 1965). What these investigations and clinical-empirical works with psychotic children demonstrate is the weight that the immediate environment of a subject plays in the psychic structuring. The mother and child relationship does not seem to be able to exclude the role of a third player, whose physical presence does not seem essential, but its discursive presence allows a necessary separation from the encroachment of an all-pervasive maternal object.

However, an absent maternal object with a non-existent father, either due to a lack of physical presence or a lack of Symbolic and Imaginary status, can also hold a stake in the formation of a psychotic structure. The case of Lefort's *Robert* embraces a very striking example of child neglect and its possible subjective and psychic consequences. Abandoned by his father and neglected by a psychotic mother, who ends up also abandoning him at 11 months of age, he passes through more than 25 different institutions and hospitals that host him without ever placing him in foster care. The massive psychotic phenomena, at three years of age, are quite manifest, and Lefort will have to deal with a very complex case (Lacan, 1953–1954; Lefort and Lefort, 1988).

5.2. The interrelationship with the parents in the assumption of the subject: castration in the case of little Hans

Little Hans's case of phobia is also of great interest for the proposal offered a few years later in *On a question prior…*, since in this case Lacan observes the Oedipal relationship between little Hans and his mother in the formation of a phobic reaction (Freud, 1909). It serves as means to make a clinical distinction between the experiences of a neurotic child with a phobic reaction, and the anxiety and psychotic productions of children like Dick or Robert. Lacan insists that the Oedipus supposes the implementation of a game in which the presence of someone is given to play that game in order to win it. The child plays the card of the one who can win the seduction game and keep the mother, it is he who possesses the real penis, even taking himself for the mother's phallus, for the cause of her desire (later in the chapter I will indicate what the phallus refers to for Lacan). Hans poses himself as a lure to the mother's desire, but especially as that which would complete her own lack, and she consents to that seduction to a certain degree by allowing him to stay in bed at night, to display his sex in front of her, etc. However, this game implies having to play with the absences and presences of the maternal object and the entrance of the father, which sets an aggressiveness in the imaginary plane. This entails a conflict of the "it's either him or me" type, which is sought to be tempered by the introduction of that Law through castration. Now this castration, Lacan reminds us, is of an Imaginary object of the body, of a fantasy type but which has symbolic effects, "a symbolic indebtedness, a symbolic castigation inscribed into the [S]ymbolic chain, and as something that snatches hold of this [I]maginary object as its instrument" (Lacan, 1956–1957, p. 211). Castration is the intervention of the Real father[1], but accomplished through the mediation of a Symbolic one, who enters the game through the prohibitions he establishes. In the case of Little Hans, his anxiety and subsequent phobia of going out into the street and being bitten by a horse were related to a moment when he was confronted with the drive, with the fact of having to show something of himself to the maternal Other, to participate in the game of seduction. The drive becomes something disturbing that thrusts him into the mystery of the Other's significations, of the mother's desire. "What invariably happens is not merely that the child simply fails in his attempts at seduction… or that he is rejected by the mother. The decisive factor is that what he ultimately has to present is something that seems to him to be something quite meagre" (Lacan, 1956–1957, p. 219), not enough. Later in the Seminar, Lacan will compliment this idea by saying: "What is called anxiety hinges on the fact that he is able to gauge the full difference that lies between what he is loved for and what he is able to give" (Lacan, 1956–1957, p. 236). Lacan even hints at Hans's confrontation at that moment in the order of sexual jouissance, although by Seminar 4 Lacan had not yet postulated the concept of jouissance. However, Freud himself suggests that there is an "exciting cause" behind this phobic reaction. Thus, for Hans it's both being unable to satisfy and fulfill the Other with a plentiful, all-encompassing gift and, at the same time, dealing with the confusing experience of the sexual drives.

In Hans, the Symbolic father operates through the intermediary of a Real father, and the effect of castration crystallizes in the fantasy narration of the plumber who comes to unscrew his widdler (*Wiwimacher*) in order to put back a new one. A fantasy in three moments, first in which he affirms that his penis is *fixed in*, that is when the phobia arises; second, when the *boring of a hole* that appears in a dream or when he decides to pierce a hole in a doll is mentioned; and finally, a third phase, is a *mediation* in which the phallus appears as something removable, which can be put on and then taken off, hence the plumber's fantasy. This emerges as a kind of resolving myth, a truth in the form of fiction. That is, the phallus is something symbolic, that nobody really possesses, which can be mobilized and combined, circulating and acting as a mediator, a signifying mediator.

5.3. The operation of myth in childhood

The proposal around Lacan's concept of myth rehabilitates the childhood theories of sexuality that Freud (1905) expounded in his *Three Essays on the Theory of Sexuality*. In other words, Hans's and children's fantasies about their place in a family, their relationship to the parental couple, their sex, their place among siblings, in a genealogy, lineage, etc., play the same role as a myth, *i.e.*, as a fiction that gathers "a singular relation to something that is always implied behind it, and which even carries within it its formally indicated message, to wit, a singular relation to truth. [...] Truth has a structure, so to speak, of fiction" (Lacan, 1956–1957, p. 245). Lacan clears out from the case of Hans the "mythemes" or the basic units that play in the Oedipus and Castration complex for this child. The myth is a symbolic expression insofar as it accounts for the mental structure organized by the environment and the original ways in which the child has to deal with the aporias that he stumbles upon. In this mediation, the neurotic child finds a way out of these impasses.

> This necessitates the integration of a fact that is already given, the fact that the mother is already an adult and that she is taken up in the system of symbolic relationships in which inter-human sexual relationships have to be situated. The child himself has to take this path. He has to experience the Oedipal crisis and its essential moment of castration. This is what the example of little Hans illustrates, but perhaps neither completely nor perfectly. It is perhaps in this incompleteness that we can find the hardest evidence of what I have indicated as the essential movement of the observation.
>
> This is a privileged case of analysis in that the transition from the imaginary dialectic can be seen being produced out in the open. We can see the child passing from this intersubjective game with the mother around the phallus to the game of castration in the relationship with the father. This passage occurs through a series of transitions that are precisely what I have called the *myths* that little Hans creates.
>
> (Lacan, 1956–1957, p. 266)

Hans, unlike children who manifest a symbiotic psychosis, experienced a decisive encounter within his Oedipus that allowed him to assume his symbolic indebtedness and his loss of jouissance through a relationship with the signifier that was offered to him by the Other. His passage through phobia was important to access this castration, hence Lacan would have suggested that phobia is a "turntable" that pivots the subject towards one of the neuroses: obsessive or hysterical (Lacan, 1968–1969, p. 307). He believed that passing through phobia is necessary for the articulation of a neurotic structure. This clearly shows the defensive mechanism of repelling the desired object, revealing it in a barely veiled way and prompting the subject to initiate a specific defense against the anxiety and unbearable nature of the object: in this case, a repressive and substitutive disguising of it.

5.4. Formalizing the first operation of lack, the original repression...

Based on the previous chapters and my discussion of the case of Little Hans, I will now propose a set-theoretical formalization of the two necessary operations of the structural lack. We move from Lacan's empirical and clinical proposal to a logical one. The first lack is universal ($\forall$), thus necessary, the second is existential ($\exists$), thus contingent. With what we have seen so far, we can write the first operation of lack.

Operation 1: $\forall_{\$}\exists_{\varnothing}$: $[\varnothing \subset \{A\} \leftrightarrow \varnothing \subset \$ \leftrightarrow \varnothing \in \{\varnothing\}]$.

This can be read as: "For every subject, there exists an empty set such as it is included in Language, if and only if (iff) the empty is included in the subject, and iff the empty belongs as an element to the empty set".

Following the axiom of empty sets, proposed by Zermelo-Fraenkel set theory, supposes a negation as its coextensive result:

$\exists_{A}$ $[\exists_{x}$ $(x \notin A)]$: "There exists an A such as there exists a null x that belongs to it".

This negation is the *Urverdrängung*.

The first operation is universal, but not the second one. From the first operation on, the toddler can start symbolizing. And it will symbolize, as described in Chapter 3, the presences and absences of the mother (or main caregiver), how "she comes and goes". What meaning should one give to those comings and goings of the mother? Only the entrance of the father (or the one that replaces him), as a function, supposes for the toddler an answer to that question. What does my mother want besides me? The toddler begins to understand the meaning of the words, that it is named, mentioned in conversations, called upon, commanded, etc., without being able to do much in the face of that "alleged omnipotence" of the Other. It will have to adjust to being a signifier, under a proper name in the {A} that the Other uses in different moments and contexts. The child quickly appraises that its introduction to the signifier supposes beginning to belong as an element of {A}, as a multiple counted-as-one marked by {ø} and questioned as something that is not included or excluded from {A}. The Other, who represents {A}, initially appears to satisfy the toddler's needs, respond to its cries, and understand its tantrums. However, the toddler soon realizes that this is not the case. The Other does not know what the toddler needs or the purpose of its tantrums. The child begins to realize that it does not truly belong to {A}, but it has no choice other than relying on it. The infant can only navigate this situation by surfing the double tension of using and being used by {A}. Caught in this drift of meaning between what the Other desires from it and what it desires of that Other but that it can fulfill or satisfy, the toddler is confronted with a second structural operation established by the Other, which implies its *aphanisis* and separation.

There must be an object beyond that evident desire of the mother, since that desire is inside a symbolic world on which she depends, and that "permits a degree of access to the object of her desire" by being "marked with the necessity the symbolic system institutes" (Lacan, 1957–1958, p. 166). Lacan will call this object the phallus (designated by the lowercase letter phi φ, as Imaginary, and the uppercase phi Φ when it is the signifier), and its negativization as what does not belong to the presentation or is an unspecularisable object of the body's image, which does not show because negativized (-φ).

This signifier implies the desire of the Other, ultimately the image of oneself and the desires of one's parents in relation to oneself ("the desired image is the image of the child that is valued by the parents and that the child comes to value as well, the child coming to value and desire what the Other values and desires" (Fink, 2004, p. 136)). Nonetheless, it is a signifier that must be lost. This is why Φ figures as the signifier of the lack in the Other, S(Ⱥ). We can then say that Φ covers S(Ⱥ); it comes to take its place without being equal to it.

5.5. ...and the second operation, castration and the Paternal Metaphor

The Φ is "chosen as the most salient of what we grasped in sexual intercourse [*copulation*] as real, as well as the most symbolic, in the literal (typographical) sense of the term, since it is equivalent in intercourse to the (logical) copula" (Lacan, 1958, p. 581). That is, Φ acts as a copulative term beyond Lacan's pun. The copula, in linguistics, is usually a word or phrase used to join the subject of a sentence with the complement of subject or adjective, or the conjunction that allows the link of two phrases. So, the copula is usually a verb accompanied by a qualifier. Before the latter quote, Lacan had stated that "the phallus is the privileged signifier of this mark in which the role [*part*] of Logos is wedded to the advent of desire" (Lacan, 1958, p. 581). The phallic signifier favors the wedding of language with desire, it is the attributive and qualitative value that allows us to capture what becomes of the object of the sexual relation, this is, as an elusive feature, which appears as hidden, but appetizing, alluring, the cause of desire.

The φ shows up as something purely Imaginary, even fantasized, which is not presented as a material object but as merely projected onto a three-dimensional plane. Some aspect of one's and the Other's body image does not reflect in the Other (three-dimensional) or the mirror (bi-dimensional), and is left outside of its constitution as unity. The – φ is left like a residue, a leftover of which the subject has no notice, scaping its awareness of body image but at the same time enshrining the body's consistency in its own incompleteness; thus, this lack is structurally necessary (Lacan, 1962–1963, lecture III; Lacan, 1960a). How is this observed in the clinic? Once again, Lemaire brings some exemplary illustrations by indicating that children's fantasies and dreams carry this castration complex and this idea of something from which he or she is separated. This implies the experiences of the lived body, the affections, the passivity, the activity, or the will to power among the experiences of jouissance, pleasure-unpleasure, and conceptual twists (Lemaire, 1977; Cavell, 1996). The castration complex figures in Lacan's Imaginary register as

> the instability with which roles and modes of being are sought to compensate... for the profound ill of human incompleteness. [...] In short, the Imaginary is

> everything in the human mind and its reflexive life which is in a state of flux before the fixation is effected by the symbol, a fixation which, at the very least, tempers the incessant sliding of the mutations of being and of desire.
>
> (Lemaire, 1977, p. 61)

In the first stage of the Oedipus complex, the toddler will seek to be that missing phallus of the mother, that object of her desire. In a second moment, the instance of the Father will be the one who deprives that phallus, not the toddler's, but the mother's. The Father's law comes into operation as a depriver of the mother, a law that does not belong to her. In a third moment, that Father ceases to be that devastating figure and who, possessor of the phallus, makes it circulate as an object of the mother's desire. "The father is the signifier in the Other that represents the existence of the locus of the signifying chain as law. He places himself… above the signifying chain" (Lacan, 1957–1958, p. 180). The conclusion of the Oedipus complex arrives at this moment, the third stage, when the identification with the father occurs, with the formation of the ego-ideal and the installation of the superego. Lacan formalizes this entire process of the Oedipus in his "paternal metaphor" (Lacan, 1957–1958, lectures IX and X); for him, ultimately, what happens in the Oedipus is a symbolic process, or has effects on the uses of the signifier and the subject-positions ($) in relation to the lack.

$$\frac{\text{Name-of-the-Father}}{\text{Desire of the mother}} \quad \frac{\text{Desire of the mother}}{\text{Signified to the subject}} \longrightarrow \text{Name-of-the-Father} \quad \frac{\text{A}}{\text{Phallus}}$$

The Oedipus complex is a metaphorical process because it consists of the substitution of the mother's desire for that of the signifier NotF. As a result of this operation, the phallus is what comes as meaning or response to the enigmatic desire attributed to the mother. This means that the father comes into play by forming a triangle where only mother and child were. However, he comes to establish himself as a father insofar as he is legitimized and called a father, as such, and to whom that function will later be attributed. The paternal function, in a nutshell, "is a requirement of the signifying chain" (Lacan, 1957–1958, p. 165).

It is in the second stage of Oedipus when the father appears as castrator and symbolic castration operates, that is, in the first stage where the mother's speech and desire represented a brute presence, now those of the father come into play through the words of the mother.

> What is essential is that the mother establishes the father as mediator of what lies beyond her law and her capriciousness—namely, the law as such, purely and simply. It is therefore a question of the father qua Name-of-the-Father, closely tied to the declaration of the law….
>
> (Lacan, 1957–1958, p. 174)

Years later, at the Seminar *R.S.I.*, Lacan would make a provocative statement: "a father does not have the right to respect, but to love only if that love is...perversely oriented, that is, directed towards a woman, the object *a* of his desire" (Lacan, 1974–1975, lecture of January 21, 1975).

The signifier NotF, mediated by the mother, supposes the maximum action that leads to castration, which, as Lacan indicated, is on an Imaginary object but establishing the lack in the Symbolic: it furnishes a law of speech and desire (NotF) whilst forcing the loss in the Symbolic (Φ). This castration is constitutive and is precisely that which is not carried out in psychosis due to the lack of the signifier NotF (Lacan, 1959).

Therefore, a second operation may or may not follow the first one,.but this time it will be a privation rather than a negation. Thus, the Other must come into play as an agent, as a third party, to generate this lack in the subject. This new actor is the Real father. The result of this operation of deprivation is S(Ⱥ). From this deprivation, we can deduce the second operation of lack:

Operation 2: $\exists_{\$} \forall_{A}: [S(\not{A}) \in \{A\} \leftrightarrow S(\not{A}) \in \$]$, under the condition that:

$$S(\not{A})=\sqrt{-1} \leftrightarrow \forall_{x} [x \in S(\not{A}) \leftrightarrow x \in \sqrt{-1} \leftrightarrow x \notin ø]$$

This second operation can be read as: "There exists at least one subject for any language, such that the signifier of the lack in the Other belongs to the set of Language iff the signifier of the lack in the Other belongs to the subject," under the condition that "the signifier of the lack in the Other is equal by extension to the square root of minus one, iff for all x, x belongs to what designates the signifier of the lack in the Other, iff x belongs to what is called the square root of minus one, and iff x does not belong to the empty set".

5.6. A formalization of the non-operation in psychosis

In psychosis, inspired by the case of President Schreber, Lacan stipulates that it is the Symbolic function of the Father, between the message and the code, that is foreclosed. Using as an example two types of hallucinations, Lacan deduces this foreclosure. On the one hand, there are the voices that speak the fundamental language to Schreber, they teach him the code, and a second group of voices that tell him how a group of messages are in the new code, which opens him to a new world of the signifier. On the other, the second type of hallucination is interrupted messages, barrages, and orders; as long as code and message are dissociated, they appear as impersonal messages or made up of neologisms.

> That's what the intervention of father's discourse resolves into, when what makes discourse coherent—namely, the self-ratification by which the father, at the completion of his discourse, goes back over it and ratifies it as law—is abolished from the start and has never been integrated into the life of the subject.
>
> (Lacan, 1957–1958, pp. 188–189)

The particularity of the Real father is to deprive the mother and try to appear as the possessor of the phallus (φ). Now, this phallus is nothing more than an

Imaginary object (φ) or a signifier (Φ), a volatile, veiled, abstract, missing object that no one really possesses. Or, it is only a supposed signifier in the Other but that is only represented in human cultures as a symbol that denies the lack, that covers it. Let us recall Lemaire's epigraph with which this chapter opened: "symbolization is human… which implies from the start: imperfection, reduction, arbitrariness, submission to external constraints and a partial failure to recognize its own mechanisms". Human symbols veil that which they cannot express, or that which the incompleteness of language cannot provide or capture. This is so deeply ingrained in language and speech that it can be seen in ancient myths. For example, in the Sumerian and Babylonian creation and heroic myths, such as *Enuma Elish* and the *Epic of Gilgamesh*, which Genesis draws heavily from, the possession of a unique, phallic-like attribute leads to disputes and tensions between the gods, resulting in wars, conflict, and epics. This signifier can be materialized, such as the "tablet of destinies", delivered by Tiâmat to his son Kingu, awarding him the gift of being able to decree the fate of any being and destroy the rival gods; a tablet that ends up being stolen from its initial owner, the god Enlil, who was never really its owner. It is a phallic signifier that circulates among the gods but that they all end up losing, no one really can grab hold of it and the power it presupposes. Who really embodies that phallic aura, that invisible power, which will favor the offerings of the faithful and the fear of the wicked?

Precisely, Φ figures as the signifier of the lack in the Other, S(Ⱥ). Lacan even indicates that – φ can be equated with the √-1, the function of a missing signifier (Lacan, 1960, p. 697). We can then say that Φ is the semblance that covers S(Ⱥ); it comes to take its place without being identical with it.

In Seminar 10, *Anxiety*, Lacan speaks of a commitment of the body in a signifying dialectic where something is separated off it, something is sacrificed, the pound of flesh that has to be delivered and projected into the Other (Lacan, 1962–1963, p. 219; Londoño, Gil, and Marín, 2023). This separation is, for Lacan, something structural that necessarily implies an agent that "extracts" or "cuts off" that pound of flesh. Some sort of symbolic act must be overcome. In this, the rites of passage of certain indigenous cultures are quite illustrative of the contingency of castration as a means to accede to a symbolic commitment (Bettelheim, 1954).

This severed object will receive a more generic designation by Lacan, object petit *a*. The phallus is a signifier, but the object *a* is unsignifying, uninterpretable, Real. It is attached to an erogenous zone, and through castration and enculturation reduced to the main orifices of the body through which the link with Other is possible. Thus, it can be related to different bodily functions, *i.e.*, all of Freud's drive objects: oral, anal, phallic, genital, and, Lacan would add, scopic and vocal (Lacan, 1962–1963, lectures XVI–XXIV). Of course, this object is mainly Real, in Lacan's sense, thus, imperceptible, supposed, unnamable beyond its technical designation (oral, anal, etc.), pure jouissance tied to erogenous zones and the experienced body.

Out of this second operation of castration, we can outline a formula for the psychotic subject:

$$\exists_{\$} \forall_{A}: [\Phi \wedge \text{NotF} \notin \$ \leftrightarrow \Phi \wedge \text{NotF} \notin \{A\}] \rightarrow \neg S(Ⱥ)$$

The non-inscription of both signifiers (Φ *and* NotF) in $ and {A} leads to the fact that the lack in the Other is lacking, negated, and more than negated, foreclosed. This means never returning as a part of the Symbolic and Imaginary registers. What corresponds to this Law that promotes the normalization of desire and the ordering of discourse? Both Φ and NotF are minimal structural forms of Language and of speaking beings, belonging to and not belonging to {A}. However, how these signifiers will be accommodated to social discourses is the result of Western Judeo-Christian culture, as I will show in Part 2 of the book.

Note

1 The Real father is a somewhat ambiguous and difficult concept to grasp in Lacan's work. In Seminar 4, *The Object Relation*, when he employs it, he seems to refer to the flesh-and-blood person who is called a father or to whom this function is attributed. In lecture XIII of this Seminar, he claims in relation to the Imaginary father that he "is a terrifying father with whom we are acquainted, who is behind so many neurotic experiences, and who bears no mandatory relation to the child's real father" (Lacan, 1956–1957, p. 212). Then, taking up the previous idea, he insists, "[w]e frequently see cropping up in the child's fantasies a figure of the father—and also of the mother—who twists into a grimace and who is very far removed from the real father who was present for the child at the time" (Lacan, 1956–1957, p. 212). The Real father has always been something difficult for the child to apprehend, precisely because of the difficulty that the knotting of the Imaginary and the Symbolic prevents it from grasping, but the concept always refers to the flesh-and-blood person in the place of the father. In the same Seminar, the Imaginary father alludes to any reference to the dialectic of aggressiveness, identification, and idealization in which that figure is involved. "It's easy to recognize that the imaginary father is the all-powerful father. This is the grounding of the world in the commonplace conception of God, the guarantee of universal order. All things real and physical, the Lord God made them all" (Lacan, 1956–1957, p. 267).

In Seminar 17, Lacan redefines the Real father as a structural operator, an agent of castration, an effect of Language, an impossibility, or the spermatozoon. He no longer sees the Real father as a specific flesh-and-blood person, but rather as an operator or a number. In Seminar 18, he asserts that the murder of the father in Freud's myth of the primal parricide is the number 0, the beginning of the count and the signifying chain. Lacan insists that the Real father is the agent of castration. However, here the word "agent" should not be taken literally as someone who performs an action. Instead, it refers to an intermediary, such as a "master agency", "my agent", or someone who is paid to do something on one's behalf. It is important to note that the Real father is more a "construction of Language" or an "effect of Language" than anything else (Lacan, 1969–1970, p. 127).

Seminar 17 will question Freud's mythical approach to the father in *Totem and Taboo*. Castration is not only a symbolic process; the Real is the logical impossibility of the Symbolic, it bores a fathomless hole in it. This idea will chain in this Seminar with Freud's castration complex, which Lacan argues is too narrow. Castration goes beyond the establishment of the paternal metaphor, where something pushes towards the necessary establishment of the Law: the regulation of jouissance. One dimension of castration falls under a structural idea, not simply an existential but a universal one, contrary to what I have argued in this chapter. Lacan will broaden the scope of the concept of castration in Seminar 17, but for practical purposes in Chapter 5, I will limit myself to the definition of Real father and castration complex from Seminars 4 and 5, unless I state otherwise.

Part 2

A genealogy of *The Father* and the Death of the Father

A quest through jouissance and Modernity

6

The patriarchy and monotheism

An "all"-mighty God

6.1. The beginnings of patriarchy and the place of the Father: the myths of procreation and origins

In her book *The Creation of Patriarchy*, Gerda Lerner describes the historical process that resulted in the institutionalization of patriarchy in West Asia (Mesopotamia) and its gradual expansion to Western societies (a 2500-year process until the beginning of the Common Era—C.E.). This was a progression that began in religion and cosmogonies, up to economies and forms of exchange. It was especially evident in the exchange of women and the regulation of their sexuality, on the one hand, and, on the other, the enthronement of male god figures as referents of the Law. The archaic States would have been organized in the form of patriarchies, or divine paternal figures, as the starting point of power relations, rooting the first legal codes in the control of the sexuality of women but also of men, marriage, property, contractual situations, etc. The prohibition of incest was one of the first forms of law whose consequence was the commodification of women, who fell to the rank of merchandise for exchange (Lévi-Strauss, 1971). For example, of the 282 laws that made up the Hammurabi Code (1750 Before the Common Era—B.C.E.) 73 were about marriage and sexual matters. In the Middle Assyrian and the Hittite laws (1450–1250 B.C.E.) more than half of the codes were on marital and sexual matters, especially the conduct of women (Lerner, 1986).

> The prohibition of incest is less a rule prohibiting marriage with the mother, sister or daughter, than a rule obliging the mother, sister or daughter to be given to others. It is the supreme rule of the gift, and it is clearly this aspect, too often unrecognized, which allows its nature to be understood. All the errors in interpreting the prohibition of incest arise from a tendency to see marriage as a discontinuous process which derives its own limits and possibilities from within itself in each individual case. Thus, it is that the reasons why marriage with the mother, daughter or sister can be prevented are sought in a quality intrinsic to these women.
>
> (Lévi-Strauss, 1971, p. 481)

DOI: 10.4324/9781032663616-9

Sacred marriage also emerged as a widespread practice in many regions of the Near East during the second millennium B.C.E., where not only kinship ties were established but also pacts between families, clans, etc., were forged through exchange. "The primordial Law is therefore the Law which, in regulating marriage ties, superimposes the reign of culture over the reign of nature, the latter being subject to the law of mating. The prohibition of incest is merely the subjective pivot of that Law..." (Lacan, 1953a, p. 229).

The association of gods or divine figures with covenants and fertility, which were expected from marriage, were of a feminine origin; the Mother-Goddesses. Throughout Mesopotamia, religious myths about procreation and origins were accompanied by a name-giving function where "nothing exists unless it has a name. The name means existence. The gods receive their existence through name-giving, as do humans" (Lerner, 1986, p. 150). The changes in mythology seem to indicate that the relationship between signifier and signified mutated over time, signaling the instability of their continual association. For example, Lerner points to the mutation in beliefs through time that went from a concept of procreation as a spontaneous act of female fertility to creation as a conscious and reasoned act of divine figures of both sexes (or asexual). This mythology in West Asia departed from verification and witnessing of events in the world (fetishism and animism) to the possibility of "creative symbolic conceptualization" and abstraction. She argues that the origin of monotheism was the idea of an omnipotent, invisible, unrepresentable, and nameless One-God embedded in paternal masculinity and in the concept of procreation. This One-God served as a species-as-operator, a symbol that could represent an inapprehensible, infinite multiple.

One of the main questions that sustains religious systems is "Who creates life?" In Mesopotamia, for centuries, mythology portrayed the Mother-Goddess as the only source of generativity and fertility. However, with the emergence of writing and symbolic systems, the Mother-Goddess came to be assisted in her fertility by male gods or kings;

> then to the concept of symbolic creativity as expressed first in 'the name', then 'the creative spirit'. We have seen... a shift in the pantheon of gods from the all-powerful Mother-Goddess to the all-powerful Storm-God, whose female consort represents a domesticated version of the fertility goddess. It remains for the pantheon of gods to be replaced by one single powerful Male god and for that god to incorporate the principle of generativity in both of its aspects. This shift, which occurs in many different forms in different cultures, occurs for Western civilization in the Book of Genesis.
>
> (Lerner, 1986, p. 180)

Lerner argues that the advent of writing, record-keeping, mathematical thinking, and the creation of symbols allowed for the possibility of creative abstraction and naming in Mesopotamia and subsequent cultures in the region. In a similar vein, Lacan locates in the invention of writing and the use of signs an effect of meaning in the Real, of grounding what remained unknowable by means of the Symbolic and the Imaginary. In more concrete terms, this means that the written sign serves as material support for the phoneme, for the sound; but more than that, writing is for Lacan the possibility of condensing knowledge into a symbolic formula, a formula that captures something of the Real. To write down a name implies being able to employ it in multiple ways, for prayers, rituals, record-keeping, and myths. The common name carries within itself the meaning that is assigned to it, while the proper name carries with it a mark, a trace, which can be uttered, and which remains in it as pure sound, as something in common regardless of the language in which it is uttered. Writing makes the proper name endure as a statement tied to phonetic features; it attributes a certain immortality to it (Lacan, 1961–1962, December 20, 1961). Naming and imagining, rooted in the symbol, are for Lerner (and implicitly for Lacan as well) the first step to condense all those anthropomorphic figures of polytheism and animism into a One-God (Lerner, 1986). Their attributes and properties would end up belonging to the Absolute set of the One; encompassing the multiple infinite. Yahwe, in the Book of Genesis, is the absolute creator of life, shaping men and women from the dust of the ground, then inhaling through their nostrils the power of his breath, bringing them to life. "Thus, the divine breath creates, but human naming gives meaning and order" (Lerner, 1986, p. 181).

6.2. The birth of monotheism and the laws of speech

Freud dates the beginning of rigorous monotheism to around 1353–1336 B.C.E., during the reign of Pharaoh Amenhotep IV of Egypt, also known as Akhenaten. He elevated the sun god Aten to the status of sole deity for political reasons, in order to consolidate his power. He persecuted those who worshipped any other god, including Amun, and established an exclusive monotheism in which he was seen as the earthly incarnation of Aten. He also excluded myths, magic, and sorcery from the religion of Aten, as well as any pictorial representations of god (Freud, 1939).

Each of Akhenaten's predecessor pharaohs had received the name of the god Amun-Re, a hybrid deity representing fertility and the sun. Akhenaten's father had this name, as did Akhenaten himself (Amenhotep, derived from Amun). Akhenaten's father, Amenhotep III, a great follower of Aten (another aspect of Amun-Re, apparently representing the light he produces), proclaimed himself a living god and called himself "the Dazzling Aten". It is unclear whether it was for political reasons, due to the growing power of the priests of the old gods and followers of Amun in Thebes, that Amenhotep IV founded a new city, Akhetaten (now Amarna), where he built temples to praise Aten—the universal light or sunlight—proclaiming him as the only universal God. He also changed his name to Akhenaten in honor of this god. A conflict began with Amun's followers, and the deities associated with him, and, apparently resulted in establishing the first monotheistic religious system.

According to Freud, Moses would have been trained under Atenism monotheism, which he ultimately transmitted to the Jews (Freud, 1939). However, some scholars doubt whether Moses even knew who Akhenaten was, since Akhenaten's religious doctrine did not prosper and died with him, and there was no literary or systematic transmission of it. Actually, most of the constructions and writings left about his legacy were purposely obliterated; Akhenaten was a rebel pharaoh whose legacy had to be repressed. Furthermore, the timelines do not seem to match, since Moses possibly lived almost 100 years after the death of Akhenaten, at a time when the transmission of Atenism had been lost into oblivion.

Beyond the historical accuracy of Freud's claim and the question of whether Moses inherited the dogma of monotheism from Akhenaten, what is interesting is to see how the story of Akhenaten and his religion insists on something key within the patriarchal tradition of Near East cultures. Some scholars of history, like W.R. Johnson (1996), suggest that Akhenaten's Aten cult was nothing more than an extension of the deification of his father, Amenhotep III. In other words, a cult of the father was maintained under the figure of a god, with Akhenaten not only worshiping his father as a god turned human, but also himself seeking to become a god later. It is about the reification of a god based on the figure of the father.

Lacan will place the key to that One-God in its revelation to Moses, when he experienced that kind of hallucinated voice emerging from a burning bush, ordering him to save the Jewish people in his name, in the name of their God (King James Bible, Exodus 3: 2–15). When Moses replied, asking what the name of God was, the answer he received was, "*I am who I am*" (*Ehyeh asher ehyeh*), which Lacan will translate in Seminar 16 as "*I am what I is*". Where an *I* (*je*) who speaks will have an extremely important effect at the beginning of Modernity. What emerges in that voice of God to Moses is founding for Lacan, it is the pronunciation and enunciation, the naming of the {ø}, of the Thing. As an {ø} it comes to being, to count as multiple-one from the moment it is named. It is the point at which God cannot be more than *what speaks*, that what appears as a pure enunciating voice that names (itself) for the first time. That is, before naming (itself) was not, was total inexistence, something identical and not identical with itself, that is, God was *nought*. "There is no other meaning to be granted to this '*I am*' than that of being the Name '*I am*'" (Lacan, 1963, p. 79). This supposes the cultural inauguration of S_1, the master-signifier, the point of departure of the Judeo-Christian world once God names itself as the inexistent set that speaks and is. Here, the NotF is presented in its radical form, resembling a name stripped entirely from the ongoing movement in which it declares itself. Thereby, the NotF asserts itself as a pure declaration, a distinct void within the signifier.

What is interesting for Lacan, however, is that later on, after an excruciating odyssey, Yahwe will deliver to Moses the tablet of the Ten Commandments on Mount Sinai, where he is no longer an *I* that speaks as *I* (*je*), but as it recognizes the other, like a *you*, "*thou shalt only worship that who has told thee* 'I am what I is', *and thou shalt only worship him*". Lacan follows: "The underlying prelude of those commandments is the You are that appoints you as I" (Lacan, 1968–1969, p. 80). The name of God opens the possibility of a new set starting from the empty set, without the latter ceasing to be included. Lacan clarifies that the subset A, or also called $\{S_2\}$, is the set of knowledge, and as we saw in Chapter 2, $\{S_2\}$ cannot be an element either inside or outside {A}. This supposes that everything that someone enunciates through {A} will be traversed by this inconsistency and incompleteness of $\{S_2\}$. For example, in certain expressions as ordinary as "it rains", establishing the grammatical subject of the phrase is not that easy. However, the phrase stands as a locus where this grammatical subject can be represented. One can situate the speaker of the sentence as something separate from the sentence articulated to the $\{S_2\}$, as a novel signifier that enunciates a truth. In other words, the name of God allows the utterer to establish itself as the subject of the enunciation in a discourse and to state truth.

Now, for Lacan, this truth goes beyond the truth by correspondence, that is, the correspondence between what is uttered and the state of affairs in the world. It is an utterance in relation to another type of truth that is based on a "legality", within the chain of signifiers.

The introduction of the Law, represented in that tablet of the Ten Commandments, also plays a preponderant role in the way in which the speech is articulated. Although this symbolic and mythical gesture does not mean the first written legal code, it seems likely that the Covenant laws and the Ten Commandments are derived from the first written codes, Ur-Nammu (2100–2050 B.C.E.), Hammurabi (1750 B.C.E.), or the Middle Assyrian and the Hittite laws (1450–1250 B.C.E.), the latter two being revisions and amendments of the Hammurabi code whose laws were already being practiced long before they were written down. However, the biblical myth of the transmission of the Commandments at Mount Sinai ratifies a crucial moment in which the Master's discourse coalesces for the Hebrew people, and that will be followed by a series of wars and genocides for more than two centuries. These Commandments serve not only to sanction and regulate but also to unite a people under the brand of a jealous God, a God who admits no competitors.

The Commandments, "in their indestructible character... prove to be the very laws of speech [parole]..." (Lacan, 1959–1960, p. 174). They are the rules for organizing subsets in order to operate with all sorts of multiples, be they material or immaterial, counted-as-one or formed-into-one-as-name inside any possible proposition stating truth. Ultimately, however, this proposal of the Commandments of God is applied in the sense that they are the ones that uphold the truth, an ideal point, a point even where the truth emerges as moral truth (Lacan, 1957–1958; 1968–1969). They regulate a separation and distancing from the Thing—"insofar as that distance is precisely the condition of speech, insofar as the ten commandments are the condition of the existence of speech as such" (Lacan, 1959–1960, p. 69).

These Commandments, at least in the Western world, extend the dimension of our conscious and unconscious actions and are the basis for the functioning of unconscious repression. Lacan seeks to make a detailed summary of these Commandments in lecture VI of Seminar 7, *The Ethics of Psychoanalysis*. This analysis stresses their civilizing character by keeping the chaos of the encounter with the Thing and the detachment from the One at a distance. Precisely the deontic dimension of the Commandments and the codes, which furnishes them, is situated in the fact that the pleasure principle is what appears as the horizon and vanishing point where *das Ding* is located. Grounded on this dimension, the subject puts in motion its distancing with respect to the Thing as a source of good (*Wohl*) via pleasure, as a source of access to a desire. Deontic practices are forged in the articulation with desire, and the first form of desire is, for psychoanalysis, necessarily incestuous in origin. The distance that Lacan considers as arising between the subject and the object originates in proximity, or with a close relative, in this case, the *Nebenmensch* that embodies the Thing. The most anxiety-producing and uncanny object is no inanimate or dangerous instrument but the fellow human being, exactly that first object (maternal) where the Thing resides. Thereby, the mother's desire and intentions are what reflects an abysmal unknown, an incognizable aspect of this object for the toddler.

Now, this close-by fellow being is both good and bad, following the Melanie Klein logic of good breast/bad breast. That is to say, the object with which, in its proximity, the toddler has access to forms of satisfaction and pleasure is also a source of unpleasure and dissatisfaction; as a matter of fact, the first source of anxiety.

> Although it must be said that at this level *das Ding* is not distinguished as bad. The subject makes no approach at all to the bad object, since he is already maintaining his distance in relation to the good object. He cannot stand the extreme good that *das Ding* may bring him, which is all the more reason why he cannot locate himself in relation to the bad. However much he groans, explodes, curses, he still does not understand; nothing is articulated here even in the form of a metaphor. He produces symptoms, so to speak, and these symptoms are at the origin of the symptoms of defense.
>
> (Lacan, 1959–1960, p. 73)

At this point, defense mechanisms against anxiety such as metaphor, substitution, displacement, projection, and others emerge as linguistic recourses, and something more fundamental, that which Lacan calls "lying about evil", is set into motion. This involves distorting a truth about desire. The defense consists of telling oneself a lie that is only revealed as such retroactively, as in the case of Freud's *proton pseudos* of hysterical symptoms (Freud, 1895; Lacan, 1959–1960). When ethical principles are imposed on consciousness or even surge preconsciously, they take the form of a commandment, like the propositions of the Ten Commandments. The reality principle emerges through the repeated imposition of ethical principles. This constant "returning to the same place", this repetition, is what structures social bonds, kinship ties, and the laws of exchange. In other words, all the discursive institutions that transform the subject into a sign, an object, or a unit within a regulated system and are fixed within the unconscious are built on this repetition. "That which over generations has presided over this new supernatural order of the structures is exactly that which has brought about the submission of man to the law of the unconscious" (Lacan, 1959–1960, pp. 75–76). However the problem of ethics begins from the moment the subject questions what is good and what is appropriate in social bonds.

Now, these commandments unfolding the whole ethical principles and the frictions between the pleasure and reality principles do not necessarily refer to any type of grammatical or syntactic law, but to an apophantic and deontic commitment, a commitment with truth. The Commandments fit effortlessly into a minimal form and structure of imperative statements; without requiring a narrative or a necessary historical or mythical support in order to operate. The Ten Commandments

> set forth the place of the subject in the nexus of prohibition and desire in speech. The decalogue itself... presents a template of the subject's primary alienation by a master signifier, the institution of the rule of speech at the expense of the idolatrous pleasures of the [I]maginary, and the traumatic production of libidinal objects that overcharge the social relation with the insufferable pressure of the drives.
>
> (Reinhard and Reinhard Lupton, 2003, p. 72)

Culture operates as a framework for the exchange of goods, upheld by myths and traditions. Conversely, religion illuminates the concealed controversies, which can disrupt or impede this flow of social and sexual interactions. Hence, religions occupy a pivotal position at the edges of the cultures in which they are ingrained. If the previous quote counts, it is because fundamental epistemic and metaphysical necessities always tend to attribute knowledge of the Real to a multiple-one and/or supernatural or mythical entity (be it in fetishistic, monotheistic, or polytheistic religions). This figure has traditionally been coextensive with the one who incarnates the Master (the king, the priest, the Dominion, the shaman, the father, the chief, etc.). They are the laws that sustain the truth of speech and pleasure as long as discourse furnishes the margins of jouissance and desire. These Commandments are prescribed by God following, in principle, no rationale, but they juxtapose prohibition and desire. This is because these laws entail the superegoic demand to take the reins of jouissance and social behavior, while they expose the imperative demand, "*Enjoy!*" They put side-by-side the tensions of the pleasure and the reality principles, the preeminence of constant aporia avowing the lack-of-being for the speaking subjects.

6.3. An "all" and a "not-all" God

The God of Judeo-Christianity is the condensation of the aporia confirmed in any deistic conception of a mythical figure inside any sort of group of speaking beings. In this sense, myths and mythologies seek, as Lévi-Strauss (1963) pointed out, to bring into play oppositions of Language, to find a possible reconciliation, a "logical model capable of overcoming a contradiction (an impossible achievement if, as it happens, the contradiction is real)" (Lévi-Strauss, 1963, p. 229). The idea of God is traversed by a dichotomy that the analyst and philosopher François Regnault (1985) recognized as an "all" and a "not-all" (*pas-tout*) god at the basis of monotheism[1]. On the one hand, between an absolute, eternal, perfect, omniscient, and omnipotent god, there is the *ens realissimum*. On the other, there is a master, Lord, king, father. The first implies The Set of all sets, it is an absolute god, the "everything", self-engendering and self-contained, an S(A), where the A appears totalized, not crossed out. The second characterizes a god who does not rule over everyone, who is not worshiped by everyone, jealous and vengeful, therefore, "not-all", who requires the other, its allegiance and recognition in order to be, thus a lacking god, S(A̸).

Now, in what we could call the "Judeo-Christian imaginary" the figure of the Antiquity's Father is associated with that of the king and God. Lacan asks these questions in his Seminar *Transference*: "Starting when, did the God of the Jews become a father? Starting when in history? Starting when in the prophetic tradition?" (Lacan, 1960–1961, p. 283). Could it be that Freud, perhaps asking himself the same questions, decided to, as a child lacking answers, create his own answer in the guise of a myth? Thus, the tyrannical Father of the primal horde in *Totem and Taboo* (Freud, 1913, pp. 141–144) and the god of *The Future of an Illusion* (Freud, 1927) describe a deity derived from the father figure, yet they are also omnipotent supernatural characters. They are the inventive fruit of Man due to his own lack, to his helplessness and impotence, to the dangers of nature and fate, and the threats of human society (Freud, 1927, p. 18). The father of the primal horde is an "all" father, uncastrated, without any limits who allows himself any jouissance, ranging from the abuse of the women of the clan to that of his own children whom he can castrate, murder, expel, etc. He is the prototype of a "potent" male figure without any weakness or flaw. This figure traverses all human mythology[2], as a signifier of the inexistent that borders on the Thing and its distressful emergence. For Lacan, the "all" and absolute Father-God (between human and divine figure) corresponds to a structural operator, to a logical necessity observed as the starting point, as 0, as seen in Chapter 1, that is, "identical and non-identical with itself", which is required to initiate the count, or its *ex*-istence—that is, that it only derives its being from an *outside* that is not (Lacan, 1969–1970, p. 123; Lacan, 1971, pp. 175–176; Lacan, 1971–1972, pp. 116–117).

However, opening a parenthesis, Lacan considers that this operation of value 0, which he identifies with the Oedipus complex in Western societies, would not be the reflection of patriarchalism. One should not seek to portray the Oedipal operation with a consubstantial form of domination or establishment of power relations between the sexes based on the masculine figure of the father. On the contrary, "it shows us how castration could be tightened in a logical approach, and in a way that I will designate as being numeral. The father is not only castrated, but precisely castrated to the point of being only a number" (Lacan, 1971, pp. 173–174). The Master's discourse that runs through millennial patriarchalism is not discarded or even denied by Lacan. The submission and exploitation of women by men, their exclusion from roles and functions that guaranteed a place in the transmission of knowledge and symbols, became institutionalized factors since the rise of monotheism (Lerner, 1986). However, what Lacan seeks here, and as the title of the Seminar where the former quote appears, is to imply that this patriarchal discourse takes the place of a semblance (*semblant*). The entire sexual relationship, between the sexes, between the genders, is a logical impossibility that disguises an obscure, veiled truth: jouissance and the semblance of castration. This patriarchal discourse has been sustained since time immemorial by a charade, a ruse, once the master obtains knowledge and power from what the slave delivers him as a product of their exploitation, they are left with nothing. In order for this discourse to predominate, the use of violence and imposition are not justified. It thrives because it puts into play a point of break, a phallic countenance that veils a structural truth, which underlies the incompleteness of the Other, Ⱥ, an incompleteness and weakness of knowledge where lack-of-being resides (*manque-à-être*).

6.4. A dead god and the all-God of Schreber

The previous statements result in another of Lacan's dictum: castration and jouissance are that semblance, which ultimately lead to the dead father (an inexistent and unrevealed God), and it is with his death that the prohibition of jouissance is decreed. The Nietzschean proclamation of the "death of God" has been a widely-discussed topic in philosophy, particularly through the perspectives of thinkers like Heidegger. Lacan was also engaged in this debate, reflecting on the controversial statement sustained by Nietzsche. In *The Gay Science*, Nietzsche (2001) conveyed the demise of God through a mythical parable, depicting a madman who proclaimed this event to a group of people, asserting that all of humanity was responsible for God's murder. According to Heidegger, Nietzsche's declaration signifies the end of the suprasensory realm—the world of Platonic and Christian afterlife, of unchanging Ideas and ideals where "everlasting bliss" resides. This world, deemed by Christianity as the only genuine one, immune to change and appearances, comes to an end with the death of God (see Chapter 8).

> If God as the suprasensory ground and goal of all reality is dead, if the suprasensory world of the Ideas has suffered the loss of its obligatory and above all its vitalizing and upbuilding power, then nothing more remains to which man can cling and by which he can orient himself. [...] The pronouncement 'God is dead' contains the confirmation that this Nothing is spreading out.
>
> (Heidegger, 1977, pp. 61–62)

This Nothing is precisely the revelation of the non-existence of this suprasensory world, the world of the afterlife. The narrative featuring this madman loudly proclaiming the murder of God, a creationist myth of Modernity, conceals the reality that God merely serves as a prominent signifier of the law and upholder of the symbolic universe. All forms of prohibition, imperatives, commandments, and their transgressions stem from the myth's implementation, transforming God into a symbol. That "dead father" is the result of mythical and historical events, a cluster of statements that defines a Language barrier, the impossibility of harmonious relationships between the sexes and of a balanced and fulfilling coexistence between humans. "He has never been the father except in the mythology of the son... [...] Man survives the death of God, which he assumes, but in doing so, he presents himself before us" (Lacan, 1959–1960, pp. 177–178).

Now, let's bear in mind that for Lévi-Strauss (1963) the myth is reversible in time. He differentiates language by its reversibility in time and speech as non-reversible. The myth would enjoy both a reversibility and a non-reversibility, it can combine both properties simultaneously. Even if what a myth describes happened a long time ago, its pattern is nonetheless timeless. It explains within a synchronicity a diachronic transcendence. Following this anthropologist, Lacan describes the myth as something that "is what provides a discursive form for something that cannot be transmitted through the definition of truth, since the definition of truth must be self-referential and since it is only insofar as speech remains in process that it establishes truth" (Lacan, 1953, p. 407). Lévi-Strauss argues that a single interpretation cannot capture the full depth of a myth. Only by comparing multiple versions can we discern the unfolding process it reveals. Building on this idea, Lacan posits an unconscious structure that shapes every speaker, encompassing lineage, family history, and individual reference points. Despite these constraints, the subject still possesses a measure of freedom to act, the possibility of variating its own individual myth.

The myth features as untranslatable; not rooted in any specific language, it is a pure manifest form of sounds (phonemes), just as a proper name can be for any language (Grigg, 2006; Lacan, 1969–1970). Here, a question that arises is: Does the myth have its own metastructure or is it the metastructure of language itself?

Standing on these questions, dichotomy, and the power to oppose pairs, is the basis of human thought, according to Claude Lévi-Strauss in *Wild Thought*. A classifying and organizing tendency would be at the bases of "mythical thought", not of the savage but of the minimum structure of thought required for logical reasoning. As I tried to show in Chapter 2, the paradoxes of the Language set {A} and of the subject ($) come into the scene at this point with the contradictions of jouissance. The different myths, both that of Oedipus and of the parricide of the primal horde (Freud, 1913, pp. 141–144), as well as the different historical myths that compose the Old Testament, expose a logical impossibility. A point where there is no accessible reconciliation in the events narrated, and which results in jouissance that is definitively prohibited since it traces the horizon of a patent threat to the cohesion of the social fabric, but at the same time leaves latent a dissatisfaction that appears as a structural gap.

> The fact that the dead father is jouissance presents itself to us as the sign of the impossible itself. And in this we rediscover here the terms that are those that I define as fixing the category of the [R]eal...the [R]eal is the impossible. Not in the name of a simple obstacle we hit our heads up against, but in the name of the logical obstacle of what, in the [S]ymbolic, declares itself to be impossible.
>
> (Lacan, 1969–1970, p. 123)

Precisely, the "all" God is a type of mythical figure of the unbarred Other, which the psychotic subject can witness as something overwhelming and ravaging. It is a totalizing imposture against which the psychotic sees itself disarmed due to the lack of the NotF and castration. For instance, Schreber, in his *Memoirs* and in Freud's reading of them, describes an "all" God, omnipotent, who forced him to repopulate the devastated world with new human beings made out of his spirit. And who also orchestrated the soul murder plan against him and turned him into a harlot, into a sexual object at the service of a man so that, once transformed into a woman, he could abuse him (Schreber, 2000, pp. 63–66, 96). He experienced visions and dreams where he felt "the almighty power of God" (Schreber, 2000, p. 10), through the presence of his "nerves" and "divine rays". This woke up in him lubricious and "feminine" sensations, "for over a year therefore the female nerves, or the nerves of voluptuousness... had penetrated my body in great masses..." (Schreber, 2000, p. 124). A ravaging might take over, constraining him to become God's companion. However, at no time does he experience this as a relationship between two, no matter how mystical it might have been. He did not take part or feel included in that experience; God was not even felt as a companion.

The *Memoirs* offer another example of the delirious experience marked by the overwhelming force of a total and unyielding castrating Father figure:

> God's rays frequently mocked me about a supposedly imminent unmanning as "Miss Schreber"; an expression used frequently and repeated *ad nauseam* was: "You are to be *represented* as given to voluptuous excesses", etc. I myself felt the danger of unmanning for a long time as a threatening ignominy, especially while there was the possibility of my body being sexually abused by other people.
>
> [...]
>
> With this phenomenon becoming increasingly manifest in the course of time, God might have become aware that unmanning was not a way of "forsaking" me, that is of freeing Himself again from the power of attraction of my nerves. From this the idea arose to "retain me on the masculine side," but again under basically false pretenses—not in order to restore my health, but to destroy my reason or to make me demented.
>
> (Schreber, 2000, pp. 124–125)

Schreber was always oppressed, subjected to a blind and impersonal force that dragged him down. That God then appears as a persecuting entity, Real father, who can enjoy of him without limits. A force that guaranteed a universal certainty, the same as in Aristotle the celestial spheres always return to the same place. Schreber, however, tended to confuse and intermingle a God *res cogitans infinita*, the totality of things, with an anthropomorphic God, "not-all", with whom he maintained an almost erotic relationship, and who could also deceive him (Lacan, 1955–1956). The foreclosure of NotF hobbles the incompletion of an Absolute Other, or its assumption as castrated. This persecuting figure reveals the psychotic's ordeal to deal with a delocalized jouissance, untied from the phallic signifier and signifying chain in which it should be inscribed. If the Other does not show castrated, lacking, it runs as a totalized figure, as an "all"-mighty force, usually tending toward the Thing, or reducing the subject to a passive object (by exploitation, subjugation, annihilation, etc.).

Notes

1 This comes from Lacan's formulae of sexuation that Lacan began constructing since Seminar 18 to see how the Oedipus complex and the Castration complex occur for men and women. Grounded in Freud's text from 1925, *Some psychical consequences of the anatomical distinction between the sexes*, and on his statements about a constitutive bisexuality in *The ego and the id*, Lacan sought to establish how, on masculine and feminine sides, given by biological anatomy, something can be located that goes beyond that anatomy and that renders account of the difference of the sexes. Sexuation (gender identity) implies the way a subject situates its experiences of satisfaction and pleasure in regard to the phallic signifier. This phallic signifier plays a role on both sides, different for the one who stands on the male side or the female side (regardless of birth sex). Both sides suppose extreme positions: the male $\exists x \overline{\Phi x}$, which is read as "there is at least one male for whom the phallic function is not fulfilled, not castrated", this is the mythical figure of the father of the primal horde of *Totem and Taboo*, and on the female side the non-mythical, elusive, impossible, and Real radical, $\overline{\exists x}\,\overline{\Phi x}$ which is read as "there is no x for whom the phallic function is not fulfilled", this is Woman. The universal quantifier also operates on both sides. On the female side, $\overline{\forall x}\,\Phi x$, which is read "not-all x fulfills the phallic function", or "not all x undergoes castration", while on the male side "all" x fulfills the phallic function, $\forall x \Phi x$. In the case presented by Regnault (1985), the god described in the scholia of the second edition of Newton's *Principia Mathematica* is located between an omnipotent male god of jouissance, $\exists x \overline{\Phi x}$, and a female god "not-all" that fulfills the phallic function, that is, it is castrated, but not completely, this lack is not all on the phallic side. There is a point of jouissance that escapes phallic regulation and is on the side of an excess, of a surplus, the Other jouissance, $\overline{\forall x}\ \Phi x$ (see note 3 of Chapter 12).

2 It is not necessary to explore mythology to see the different figures of tyrannical kings or lords, from King Pheron, the Thirty Tyrants, Caligula, Nero, Vlad the Impaler, Gilles de Rais, or Ivan the Terrible. Although many of these historical accounts are not reliable or confirmed, they do hide behind them the shadow of this fantasy of a figure of an omnipotent male not crossed by castration, the Imaginary Father of Seminar 4.

7

God of vengeance and jouissance

A God that is "not-all"

> [...] for voluptuousness became God-fearing, and God himself (his father) never tired of demanding it from him.
>
> (Freud, 1911, p. 56)

7.1. The jealous king is "not-all": a look at the flawed God

The people of Israel, initially made up of 12 nomadic or semi-nomadic tribes, based their kinship relationships and ethnicity on their blood ties and on "responsibility for blood-vengeance" (Lerner, 1986). If someone from the family or tribe was harmed, he had to be avenged, even by killing his attacker or someone from their family. Lerner recounts how as the 12 tribes grew and became stronger, under the leadership of Joshua, after the death of Moses, they set out to conquer Canaan, a period dominated by war, rape, infanticide, and massacres of all kinds; narrated in the Bible in the book of Joshua and continued in that of Judges—but supported by the books of the Torah (Numbers and Deuteronomy). This period takes up almost two centuries of the history of the Israelites' conquest and occupation of Canaan (1270–1020 B.C.E.). In these books arises the God who commands his followers to end nations or peoples (the Canaanites and the Midianites), a vengeful God, a God of fury and rivalries. However, the books also hold in the background a God of love and kindness towards his servants and his people, but reserved only to them.

> Ye shall not go after other gods, of the gods of the people which *are* round about you; (For the Lord thy God *is* a jealous God among you) lest the anger of the Lord thy God be kindled against thee and destroy thee from off the face of the earth.
>
> (King James Bible, Deuteronomy 6: 14–15)

Another passage in the book of Nahum states: "God is jealous, and the Lord revengeth; the Lord revengeth, and is furious; the Lord will take vengeance on his adversaries and he reserveth wrath for his enemies" (King James Bible, Nahum 1: 2). This "not-all" God is a god imbued with human shortcomings, despite seeking

DOI: 10.4324/9781032663616-10

to understand the radical difference between men and God that the Book of Genesis tries to fulfill, the following books of the Bible sink deeper in a pursuit to hold close as a bearer of the Law the signifier of the Lord. If as a totalized incommensurable signifier, the people of Israel seemed not to be prey of fear over his inscrutable might by idolizing other gods, other goods, other forms of jouissance (the golden calf, for instance), appealing to humanlike trends attempted to bring closer the infidel or the skeptic. God is anthropomorphized, placed at the level of a monarch with a human appeal, and who, like any monarch, can dispose of his subjugates, punish them, expatriate them, unleash his fury, etc. He resembles a capricious, even despotic monarch, but this corresponds to men's own inherent lack, a weakness that they project onto God as a force, as a fact of their own constitutive flaw. He is the semblance of the omnipotent and foolproof patriarch. What this figure of the despot coats is a dark, destructive background inherent to the heart of the speaking being; the abysmal inscrutability of the Thing, right in the kernel of the *Nebenmensch.*

The first two Commandments of the tablets ("thou shalt have no other gods before me" and "thou shalt not make into thee any graven image, or any likeness of any thing that is heaven above, or that is the earth beneath, or that is in the water under the earth: thou shalt not bow down thyself to them, nor serve them…" (King James Bible, Exodus 20: 3–5)) exhibit certain proscriptions that break with animistic (fetishistic and totemic) and polytheistic traditions, radically separating god and man from nature. God is nothing representable on Earth, he is unnamable, "the signifier that transcends any meaning it might attract, and in the process inaugurates the signifying chain" (Reinhard and Reinhard Lupton, 2003, p. 78). This alienation of man to Language, but radically separating him from nature, is a decisive step towards Modernity and the emergence of science. Man will take himself as a measure and reference of transcendence over the things of the Earth.

7.2. Living with the ambivalence of jouissance, or how to regulate it

Judeo-Christian discourse, a set of laws, values, and symbols, continues to run through Western culture, undergirding key fantasies of personhood, nationhood, and neighborhood (Reinhard and Reinhard Lupton, 2003, p. 71). If we take what was stated at the beginning of the previous chapter plus what has just been expressed, two points stand out from this brief historical account and tradition: 1. The control of sexuality and pleasure; and 2. Violence, apparently unstoppable and unrestricted among humans, will find certain limitations based on divine laws and covenants. Behind these constitutive historical events of Judeo-Christianity hides something that Lacan will seek to emphasize throughout his entire work: the problem of jouissance. How is the unchained jouissance that prevents the formation of a culture regulated?

In his works *Civilization and its Discontents* and in *Totem and Taboo* Freud attempts to show the way jouissance is regulated, as it figures as an unnamable {ø} that inhabits the hearts of speaking beings and makes harmonious coexistence difficult.

Jouissance is experienced precisely as that which cannot be counted-as-one, and whose formation-into-one is problematic. An almost ineffable experience of one's and the other's body; traversed by tension and pleasure. It is multiple dispersed, elusive, Real, which resists symbolization and signification. Both Freud and Lacan unavoidably consider in biblical passages the Commandments within the ongoing governance of speech laws, intertwined with jouissance in a dual manner. First when God vociferates the Commandments in an anguishing and unintelligible utterance, figuring as a pure and nude invocative drive object. Thus, as a rumble incarnating a superegoic jouissance. And second, the tablet of the Commandments and Moses uttering them one by one to the Hebrew people where their imperative character persists even nowadays within the social Western organization of society (Reinhard and Reinhard Lupton, 2003).

What Lacan catalogs as the "ferocious ignorance of Yahwe" in Seminar 17 supposes that this is a god who ignores everything about other religions and other gods, but above all, who ignores everything about sexuality, about sexual knowledge. The Sumerian and Babylonian gods who fertilized the world, or who in their copulation brought fertility, abundance, creation, etc., are something unknown to Yahwe since he himself is self-engendered and outside any natural world, outside of the signifier. This inaugurates a new discourse, the Master's discourse, founded on the first two Commandments and Yahwe's jealousy. "The Master inaugurated by Judaism repudiates pagan pan-sexualism, knows nothing about sex, yet continues to embody a disturbingly violent element of jouissance, precisely through the ferocity of that ignorance" (Reinhard and Reinhard Lupton, 2003, p. 81).

These first two Commandments seek to keep away any other signifier that could generate another meaning apart from the non-dialectable and unquestionable commands of not loving pagan gods or idolizing them. It is the full assumption of a nascent monotheism where religion, in addition to a new legal code, emerges as something independent of the rest of the culture and its pagan and almost sinful practices. Precisely, what makes humans unique in contrast to the rest of nature is the fact of being inscribed in Language; it is what separates them from the animal world but at the same time snares them in the paradox of jouissance and the incompleteness of this Language. In this order of ideas, the Master's discourse that is founded aspires to generate a totalizing knowledge about things, but without including sexuality. Sexuality is not something that concerns God as the sole and omnipotent master, but rather it concerns men of flesh and blood, in their incompleteness and imperfection, in their weakness for the "pleasures of the flesh", or the approach of deadly jouissance. Sexual jouissance will only be accosted in the seventh and tenth Commandments ("neither shalt thou commit adultery"; "neither shalt thou covet thy neighbor's wife, neither shalt thou covet thy neighbor's house, his field or his manservant, or his maidservant, his ox, or his ass, or any *thing* that *is* thy neighbor's" (King James Bible, Deuteronomy 5: 18, 21)). The foundation of ethics occurs precisely in the link between Law and desire, and the maternal object, or the incestuous desire as the source of all desire. The objective is to keep that object of desire at a distance; "…the covetousness that is in question is not addressed to anything that I might desire but to a thing that is my neighbor's Thing" (Lacan, 1959–1960, p. 83). It is in speech that the prohibition that enunciates the need to distance oneself from the Thing is based; this is, the *thing* of thy neighbor. The Thing is only known because the Law makes it known; the covetousness is introduced because it was first forbidden as Law. Thus, we can say that that is how the beginning of the dialectical relationship between desire and Law comes into play.

7.3. The imperative opacity of the Law

Freud's myth of the primal horde parricide interpolated with a new myth of Moses in *Moses and Monotheism*, is like a myth in the sense that it is a story that maintains the structuralist perspectives proposed by Lévi-Strauss (Lévi-Strauss, 1963; Freud, 1939). Both myths seek to reconcile antagonistic positions in an unresolved conflict around a parricide, which leads to a structural antagonism: absolute jouissance vs. the impossibility of its total expression. Absolute jouissance leads to destruction and self-destruction, no jouissance at all to stagnation and no social bond. Jouissance appears as both what enables and impedes the social bond.

Jack Goody in his work, *The Logic of Writing and the Organization of Society*, shows how literate societies and those with written traditions based on a universalizing monotheism are conflicted with these aporias under the guise of "cognitive contradictions" or "cognitive dissonance" (Goody, 2001). The legal codes do not seem to be enough to avoid the overflow of jouissance, or in any case, they do not cover all the occasions of its expression or all those possibly involved in its overflow. When Commandments like "thou shalt not kill" appear to bend for specific groups or situations, contradictions abound. Even honorable wartime deaths or those from feuds (duels, slayings of honor, etc.) demand a societal forgiveness or atonement, acknowledging the inherent human cost. This same ambivalence extends to the taking of animal life. Goody posits "humanitarian feelings" as a source of this cognitive dissonance. While the term remains ambiguous, it likely points to some human condition whereby the capacity for compassion and empathy are expressed. However, delving deeper, the idea of otherness—whether animal, fellow being, or unknown—holds a peculiar intrigue. Within this difference lies a reflection of ourselves, an unknown that stirs a primal urge to bridge the gap, to access the Thing. This Thing, shrouded in endless mystery and repulsion, exerts a paradoxical pull. Like the terrifying allure of an abyss, it beckons us with invasive anguish, keeping us teetering on the edge, both repelled and inexplicably drawn in.

In this opacity of the law, we also have the case of the Hammurabi code, which enthroned the patriarchal family as the model and the minimal cell, the building block, of Mesopotamian societies and, much later, Western societies. The archaic state recognized in the ordering and regulation of the nuclear family an equivalence with the regulation and control of public affairs. For instance, in the Middle Assyrian laws, a pregnant woman who self-induced an abortion would be considered a traitor to the king and the community. According to Lerner (1986), this shows the overlap between the public power of the king (state) and the power of the patriarch over the life of his children and wife. Only the father had the right to dispose of the life of his children, not the wife, as that would be usurping an exclusive right of the patriarch. "The control of female sexuality, previously left to individual husbands or to family heads, had now become a matter of state regulation. In this, it follows... a general trend towards increasing state power and the establishment of public law" (Lerner, 1986, p. 121). However, the right to take a life, even within one's own family, could be granted under specific circumstances. This flexibility in permissible killing often coincided with an established normative code that dictated who had the right to a certain portion of jouissance and who didn't. This code determined who could benefit from the usufruct of the other's body and who was denied that right.

For Lacan, the Ten Commandments that emerge from these first legal codes have something indistinctive, something that insists as a categorical imperative on their perpetuation beyond any practical reason of their applicability and utility, such as that pursued by Kant's practical reason or Spinoza's ethics.

> The ten commandments... are tied to the deepest of ways to that which regulates the distance between the subject and *das Ding*—insofar as that distance is precisely the condition of speech, insofar as the ten commandments are the condition of the existence of speech as such. For from another point of view, how can one not in truth see, when one merely recites them, that they are in a way the chapter and verse of our transactions at every moment of our lives? They display the range of what are properly speaking our human actions. In other words, we spend our time breaking the ten commandments, and that is why society is possible.
>
> (Lacan, 1959–1960, p. 69)

The indestructible character of laws and covenants resides in their ability to protect the subject vis-a-vis the Thing. The condition of speech determines the civilizing possibilities. As Freud claimed, they maintain a double tension with respect to jouissance. This double tension evinces a Janus between barbarism and civilization, between pleasure and unpleasure, and between death and preservation of life. The revelation of God to Moses through the burning bush, disclosing its name, the Tetragrammaton (YHVH) or the unpronounceable name of God, becomes the S_1 or the main signifier, point of departure for all human affairs and creation. It silently upholds the discourse of the Other in a crucial manner by submitting the speaking subjects and denying them access to total jouissance. However, this jouissance doesn't vanish entirely but remains attached to this S_1, the Name of God and to the Thing masked by this signifier. So, the name retains this twofold quality, preserving a *plus-de-jouir*, or a surplus of enjoyment while hiding agony and suffering.

At a certain point in his work, Lacan, following *Civilization and its Discontents*, suggests that jouissance is evil [*un mal*], "it is suffering [*mal*] because it involves suffering [*le mal*] for my neighbor" (Lacan, 1959–1960, p. 184). Jouissance is the beyond of the pleasure principle, the interstice of pleasure-unpleasure; of pleasure sucked by the inevitable vacuum of the death drive, or how one can go beyond the limits of the Law, by skimming the Thing. It implies some sort of coerced automatism or repetition compulsion of a beyond-the-pleasure not necessarily tied to some biological condition. Repetition, as Freud indicated, is the return to the inanimate, to the state of zero tension, where death is the ultimate goal. It is the tendency to return towards the Thing, where death dwells as the last bastion of the impetus of repetition in the acts of life. However, jouissance is not considered by Lacan solely as an unpleasantness based on the repetition compulsion, since it also includes pleasure, as when he indicates how there is jouissance in sublimation and artistic creation. Jouissance is the way in which the body and Language find incomplete forms of satisfaction. For instance, the symptom provides a secondary gain, which the subject is reluctant to give up. Even though the symptom causes suffering, it also offers a minimal level of satisfaction, this is jouissance.

7.4. The Real father and Enuma Elish

Phallic jouissance, or jouissance of the signifier, filters into the chain of signifiers, in the statements and in how speech and meaning are concatenated. In the prohibitions conveyed by the Biblical Commandments, one can suspect the presence of that jouissance. For instance, the second Commandment, according to Jesus in the book of Matthew, apparently seeks diminishing, if not countering, that jouissance under an imperative proposition: "*Thou shalt love thy neighbor as thyself*" (King James Bible, Matthew 22: 39). This Commandment is not part of the Talmudic tradition but the main imperative introduced by Christianity: to love the *Nebenmensch* unconditionally, no matter any wrongdoing on its behalf. Jesus demands embracing our neighbor even in its most alienating and anxiety-producing incarnation of the Thing.

However, for Freud this seems impossible, not only because of the contradictory messages repeatedly coming from Father-God who asks us to love and then to avenge him with death, but because of a constitutive narcissism belonging to any speaking being and to its batch of jouissance that it is not so easily willing to give up to anyone. To love someone who doesn't merit it or that has no basis for some reciprocal fondness seems impossible (Freud, 1930).

> ...Freud stops short in horror at the consequence of the commandment to love one's neighbor, we see evoked the presence of that fundamental evil which dwells within this neighbor. But if that is the case, then it also dwells within me. And what is more of a neighbor than this heart within which is that of my jouissance and which I don't dear go near? For as soon as I go near it... there rises up the unfathomable aggressivity from which I flee, that I turn against me, and which in the very place of the vanished Law adds its weight to that which prevents me from crossing a certain frontier at the limit of the Thing.
>
> (Lacan, 1959–1960, p. 186)

Even if the Law, the second of Jesus's commandments, as a moral imperative, may vanish, it still prevents us from crossing that limit that we have been talking about, from avoiding the horror of the void that constitutes the Thing. "It is necessary to prohibit that catastrophe of presentation which would be its encounter with its own void, the presentational occurrence of inconsistency as such, or the ruin of the One" (Badiou, 2005, p. 93). The floating signifier NotF, which is settled in a myth, allows to veil the Thing and give shape to the chain of signifiers and the establishment of the laws of speech. In the patriarchy denounced by Lerner, the Father-God has fulfilled a "sublimatory function" that favors a certain "apprehension of reality as such" and a "normalization of desire" (Lacan, 1959–1960, p. 181). How does this happen? How does the Father, as a pure myth and signifier—beyond his masculinizing and excluding incarnation in the Other—open towards the apprehension of reality and a normalization of desire? A normalization, since we already saw how the Commandments arise from his voice as Law, while the name of the Father-God is S_1. And he is a father because he is established in the semblance of a patriarchal society. As for the apprehension of reality, since Freud had already suggested in *Totem and Taboo*, and later in *Moses and Monotheism*, that the function of the father is a sublimation, a novel opening towards a spirituality (*Geistigkeit*). While the idea of a primal father promoted a rejection of magic, superstition, and mysticism, in an impulse to be empowered by truth, the monotheistic religion opened for the Jewish people a new way of living intellectuality (spirituality) and morality (Freud, 1939, p. 86). In some way, then, a new form of reinterpreting the presentations and re-presentations of objects in the world and with the Other was reformulated. This primal father incarnated in Moses for the Jewish people was not just the representative of a "patriarchal civility" and the humanitarian ideal that Goody told us about, and that Freud somehow also glimpsed. However this romantic figure of an affectionate, wise, and pious father, full of love for his people depicts, it is not the way in which the establishment of the Law begins. For Lacan and Freud, it seems that there is something more substantial in what is the mythical and structural aspect of the establishment of the order of speech (*parole*), and the deontic and apophantic positions of the relationships between speaking beings. This is based on the idea of the Real father, but not the flesh-and-blood father, Real in the full sense of what this means. The Real father, as Lacan lays out in Seminar 17, *The Other Side of Psychoanalysis*, will become an impossible signifier and image to grasp, thereby the father who enjoyed all the women of the clan, or the "all" Father-God of the Old Testament mentioned in the previous chapter. He becomes the agent of castration and a logical operator.

> It is at the level of the [R]eal father as a construction of language, as Freud pointed out moreover. The [R]eal father is nothing else than an effect of language and has no other [R]eal. [...] It is the position of the [R]eal father as articulated by Freud, namely, as impossible, that makes the father necessarily imagined as a depriver. [...] It necessarily, structurally depends on something that evades us, which is the [R]eal father. And is strictly out of the question that

> the [R]eal father be defined in any assured manner unless it's as the agent of castration. [...] Castration is a [R]eal operation that is introduced through the incidence of a signifier, no matter which, into the sexual relation.
>
> (Lacan, 1969–1970, pp. 127–129)

Thus, Lacan proposes a mythical father, like that of the myth of *Totem and Taboo*, who is not unrepresentable but rather multiple, taking various forms of impasses depending on the culture and situation. The mythical father is a metonymic displacement of the God of revenge and punishment (Imaginary father), but a God who leaves behind an impossible to solve event (Real father). The Real father incarnates more a series of impeded actions and mythical events (human conflicts and discordant relationships) than some personification of a tyrannical figure, whilst maintaining this primordial signifier latently operative. Lacan suggests that we can't help but feel in our very bones the presence of those essential signifiers, the anchors without which human meaning would stray away, the mythologies sustaining them through generations. "Isn't it on the contrary clear that these mythologies are aimed at installing man, at placing him upright, in the world—and that they tell him what primordial signifiers are, how to conceive their relationships and their genealogy?" (Lacan, 1955–1956, p. 200). For instance, many things remain unresolved regarding creation itself after returning to the *Enuma Elish* creationist myth of Sumer, Babylon, and Assyria (2000–1600 B.C.E.). For instance, what created Apsû and Tiâmat, the fresh and salt waters? Where did they themselves come from? Who created the heavens and earth? Were they always there, the waters? They intermingled and conceived their children. Again, a parricide comes into place as some sort of inescapable event, in this case, the murder of the great-grandfather, Apsû, by the hands of Ea, unleashing the conflict between the gods. And later, a second parricide, that of Tiâmat at the hands of her great-great-grandson, Marduk, which puts into motion creation as such by raising an empire upon the dismembered body of his great-great-grandmother. Marduk creates from the pieces of her body the celestial vault, establishes the seasons and the abodes of the gods, the storms and the winds, and the climatic cycles, that is, the order of the world. How from two parricides, and why precisely from parricidal acts, is the order of the world given? This remains something difficult to grasp, something unanswered, but it signals the first step towards Language and civilization. A radical act, the murder of a parent, means the setting in motion of the Law. The limit imposed by this Real series of events becomes a structural need; it operates as an anchor stitch adrift of jouissance that would represent the catastrophe of the presentation, that is, the reencounter with the Thing.

Within the origin story, an inscription emerges—a mark that lays the foundation for knowledge. This inscription pierces the timeless void of pre-symbolic existence, establishing a connection between men and the father figure. Notably, this connection retroactively articulates the father within the very origin of humanity and Language itself. The symbolic murder of the primal horde represents the fracturing of the preexisting order, prompting the brothers to forge a new bond—a pivotal step in the formation of civilization.

8

Is Modernity a precursor of psychosis?

8.1. An ethnopsychiatric hypothesis

A cultural psychiatry hypothesis suggests that psychosis was settled in the patriarchal, Judeo-Christian Western world. R. Littlewood and S. Dein (2013) launched into the ocean of sociocultural hypotheses of schizophrenia the idea that the latter would have emerged at the time of the expansion and establishment of Christianity and, later, Modernity in the Western world. This is a hypothesis that is indebted to ethnopsychoanalyst Georges Devereux (Devereux, 1977). Although they do not speak from psychoanalysis but from psychology, their proposal does open a clue to look forward to what the entry of Christianity was like and what it meant, in the changes and ways of relating between members of communities, and how this favored the emergence of schizophrenic psychosis. Their argumentation tends to emphasize Modernity's individualism rather than Christianity itself, as it appears as a fruit of this Christian-made anthropological mutation, figuring as the showrunner in the metamorphosis process of Western enculturation and oppression in European colonized cultures. According to these authors, the passage to European, historical, and cultural Modernity deemed an increase in psychotic patterns. These authors suggest that there is no clear evidence and rare descriptions of what is currently understood as schizophrenia in pre-Christian civilizations. In most of the testimonies in Babylonia or ancient Egypt, madness was associated with disruptive, irrational, and impulsive behaviors. In ancient Greece there was no clear difference between madness and delirium, with even the Hippocratic corpus confusing them in descriptions where there was presence of fever and manic characters. In Greek myths and tragedies, madness was associated with extreme passions or frenzy.

In ancient Greece there was no notion of an interiority, of an ego, as such, there was no such idea of an inside and an outside of oneself, but a continuity where men felt pain or discomfort as they could feel a god, an animal, or the weather that was approaching warmly or aggressively. One's feelings were multiple, mobile, they didn't just belong to one but to the multiple. Madness was more associated with moments of intense passion, debauchery, and violent outbursts. In addition, madness was not something that belonged to one or one's interior, to the self, but rather it came from outside; it was invasive and an autonomous entity, and it could

DOI: 10.4324/9781032663616-11

even be personified in many tragedies, such as the case of Lyssa in Euripides' tragedy, *The Madness of Heracles*. Mania, as Ruth Padel explains, was not just a fit of sudden madness but a god, the god Mania, the Eumenides or the Furies, the personification of vengeance and wrath, "divinities personifying fits of *mania*" (Padel, 1995, p. 21). Madness would be a temporary loss of normal consciousness mainly provoked by the anger of a god, or because of some spell that was laid upon someone. This type of culture, psychoanalyst P.-H. Castel calls "cultures of persecution", as opposed to "cultures of guilt". In other words, the former are cultures where the moral conscience and the intimate involvement of the individual do not figure anywhere in the explanation that is elaborated on in the discontents or misfortunes that happen to that person (Castel, 2008). We will have to wait for the arrival of Modernity for this to begin to happen.

Devereux, precursor of ethnopsychoanalysis, points out that in "truly primitive" societies (primitive in the sense that their members know more and better their territory and culture of origin compared to modern humans who only know sections of their culture and territory) there is almost no evidence of cases of schizophrenia, and in those cases that are currently identified it seems to be more due to their passage through a process of Westernized enculturation. It is in Judeo-Christian Western modernity, even at the end of the fall of Rome, that cases that could be compared to schizophrenia would have been consolidated, at least as described by contemporary psychiatry (Devereux, 1977; Littlewood and Dein, 2013).

The entry into Modernity in Western Europe led to an increase in the observations of chronic cases, apparently incurable and with a poor prognosis. This does not mean that in the Middle Ages in Europe madness or folly did not exist or was not observed. However, the descriptions provided by physicians, philosophers, and historians often diverge significantly from what we recognize as contemporary manifestations of schizophrenia and hebephrenia. In the Middle Ages, medical practices largely adhered to the Hippocratic classification, maintaining categories such as mania, melancholia, epilepsy, and lethargy inherited from Greek Antiquity (Londoño, 2016). Alternatively, the perception of a mad individual was often rooted in the belief that they were either a sinner or possessed, leading to their care being entrusted to religious authorities, compassionate folks, and charity (Quétel, 2012).

One might consider whether Modernity simply brought these conditions into clearer focus, rendering them more tangible, objectifiable, and subject to the discourse of science and reason. Rather than providing a definitive answer to this question, I prefer to keep the possibility open for an alternative perspective to that proposed by Littlewood and Dein.

By Modernity I mean a process of mutation where human relationships and experiences of being in the world were based on the emergence of a new mode of encounter based on personal interiority and individuality. Following Charles Taylor, it can be deduced that from the moment the idea that each individual had a self, and more precisely, an inner moral self, we initiated a new type of society. Modernity is the historical period that saw the individual become the central agent of social events and who enjoyed a degree of autonomy and decision-making. Hence, the collectivity, the institutions and existential meaning turn around the individual or the self, and not some larger organization (the king, the feudal lord, the nation, God, etc.) or some collective purpose (glory, nations enrichment, conquest, evangelization, etc.). The human subject is rethought in relation to politics, the economy, the arts, and its place in the world, which leads to the formation of democratic and constitutional states, capitalism, science, and countless other profound changes in many areas. It signs the end of the Middle Ages and the decline of the monopoly of the Catholic Church's metanarrative over knowledge, truth, power, and libidinal economy (pleasure-unpleasure).

More precisely, Littlewood and Dein have set their sights on Christianity (mainly Protestantism) and individualism as precursors of this chronicity, and this encourages me to try getting closer to what this could mean at the NotF level. Why did the dominance of Christianity, and then the entry of Protestantism in the 16th century C.E., into the ways of life have an impact, if not in the emergence, at least in the increase of schizophrenia? Littlewood and Dein (2013) rely on the work of Louis Sass (1992, 2001) and the idea of an "excessive" reflexive self-consciousness spread by Modernity, in which the external world becomes less reliable, less a guarantor of truth, and it is only the interiority of the individual experience that must sustain the becoming, "exacerbating self-alienation". This is not very far from the Lacanian proposal of the foreclosure of the NotF signifier and of the inconsistency, even the death, of the big Other[1].

8.2. The precursors of Modernity in philosophy and religion

To begin with, the 3rd and 4th centuries C.E. brought an important figure in this process towards Modernity; Augustine of Hippo. He was considered one of the first philosophers and theologians, according to Charles Taylor in his book *Sources of the Self*, to introduce the idea of inwardness, the adumbration of the *self*, to the Western world. Distinguishing between an internal man and an external man, the external man being everything that is in common with the animal, including our senses, and our memory, while the internal man is the one who enjoys a soul. To transcend and reach God, one must have an interior (Taylor, 1989). Taylor takes up a famous phrase by this author: "Do not go outward; return within yourself. In the inward man dwells truth" (p. 129). The direct path to God is in us, and Augustine provides us with the language of inwardness, which means that he calls for self-reflexivity where knowledge is a matter of the individual in contact with its own self. It opens the path to a first-person standpoint of experiences as something crucial to higher conditions and thus a new appraisal of moral sources in Western culture. Augustine is the introducer of proto-Cartesianism by giving us a "certainty, that is a certainty for me; I am certain of my existence: the certainty is contingent on the fact that knower and known are the same. It is a certainty of self-presence" (Taylor, 1989, p. 133).

Taylor identifies self-responsible autonomy, recognized individual particularity, self-control by reason, and personal commitment to the common good as the basis of the emergence of modern individualism. The Protestant Reformation in the 16th century C.E. marked a turning point in the relationship between individuals, and with God, faith, and morality. The Catholic Church was no longer the only channel for believers to reach God. Unlike Catholicism, the Lutheran, Calvinist, and Anglo-Saxon Puritan churches placed the individual believer as the sole channel for communication with God through preaching and good deeds. For Calvinism, for example, it is only through hard work and personal responsibility that one obtains salvation. There is no mediation for its obtention as the Catholic church had established it. In Protestantism, each one must rely on one's actions, on one's deeds, and not just in one's membership in a religious community, or daily confessions and "paying indulgences" as a way out of damnation. Therefore, buying one's way out of sin through constant confession and penitence are not enough for one's absolution. Only through "wholehearted personal adhesion" to the cause or the calling can each individual become responsible for its own salvation.

> Where a mediated salvation is no longer possible, the personal commitment of the believer becomes all important. [...] I am a passenger in the ecclesial ship on its journey to God. But for Protestantism, there can be no passengers. This is because there is no ship in the Catholic sense, no common movement carrying humans to salvation. Each believer rows his or her own boat.
>
> (Taylor, 1989, p. 217)

For example, Puritanism emphasizes seeking God's glory in all things, including trivial chores and daily work. We must devote ourselves "earnestly and unremittingly" to our calling, serving God and others through hard work (Taylor, 1989, p. 224). The calling to serve is open to anyone who is willing to listen to and follow God, not just those in monastic life or the priesthood. Therefore, before the calling, we are all equal, regardless of our place in the social hierarchy. Sanctification can only be achieved through our work in the habits of daily life, which is also a way of serving God and others. This is where Max Weber saw the basis of capitalism and its discourse. Weber believed that the Puritan notion of the calling helped to foster a way of life focused on disciplined, rationalized, and regular work, coupled with frugal habits of consumption. This form of life greatly facilitated the development of industrial capitalism (Taylor, 1989, pp. 225–226).

At the beginning of Modernity, around the late 16th and the 17th centuries, these Augustinian and Protestant postulates were exalted and made available to a broad public. Highly influenced by this work ethic of Anglo-Saxon Puritanism, Francis Bacon raised the first postulates of what would become empiricism and the new science in Europe. Both Bacon and theological puritanism see the work of man as something necessary that must be fully performed for the service and benefit of humankind. Science should not be at the service of contemplation, or as a kind of epistemic curiosity, but of progress and effective productivity. The facts of the world start from efficient causes, from a mechanism, thus there are truths of faith and truths of reason. However, the observation of the facts of nature must be carried out without prejudice, taking them as they occur and are given by themselves, and it is there that the truths of reason must be located. The technical method must be based on experimentation, but this is done by overcoming the obstacles that stand in the way of scientific progress. The weaknesses of the human race are those prejudiced obstacles that he calls "idols": the idols of the tribe (accommodating our beliefs to the facts, interpreting anthropomorphically); the idols of the cave (errors and characteristic biases of each one that come from personal characteristics); idols of the forum (the social character flawed by Language); and the idols of the theater (previous ideologies and wrong philosophical systems). The approach to these idols, in his *Novum Organum*, not only questions the long logical tradition of Aristotle (*Organon*) but also comes to question all the classical conceptions of the purpose of mankind and its place in the world. Bacon (2000) seeks to break with all metaphysical speculation not based on observable facts, that is, what cannot be accounted for by inductive and experimental methods. This is an idea that would materialize with positivism in the 19th century in the hands of A. Comte and J.S. Mill. For Bacon there are no longer truths by a statute of authority, nor are there any systematizable truths, but rather cumulative ones that produce utility. Bacon's contribution is that the God of Antiquity is no longer sufficient to sustain any truth about the meanderings of the Universe. Man will have to fend for himself to collect any truth, which will now have to yield to the discourse of scientific induction and deduction, to reasoning.

The convergence between Puritanism and Baconian science not only pointed to an instrumentalization of the resources and means of nature for productive purposes and the benefit of humanity, but in the background they also sought to serve God, to preserve and increase his glory. The point is that we should treat the things of God's creation as means to pay tribute to God and help others, and not as ends in themselves. However, this idea and theological point of view of work and profit for God was lost along the way.

8.3. The cartesian turn

René Descartes is another key philosophical figure of Modernity and individualism. His work reflects the new movements of the time, particularly in its emphasis on truth and knowledge as arising from the clear and distinct presentation of things. Descartes believed that one could re-represent any presentation to oneself in an organized and rational way. To achieve this, Descartes proposed disengaging from our bodily perceptions and descriptions, which could deceive us. He suggested objectifying things and perceiving them as alien to us, functioning mechanically and independently of any teleological entity. In other words, we should approach objects "by understanding them as 'disenchanted', as mere mechanism, as devoid of any spiritual essence or expressive dimension" (Taylor, 1989, p. 146).

A key difference between Descartes and the Platonic-Augustinian tradition is that Descartes does not guarantee a divine cosmic order of the Good that sustains the soul. For Descartes, this order does not exist. There is no certainty of a divine order providing structure to matter. Instead, humans must apply reason to build that order.

Descartes definitively separates the individual from the object and makes one consider it as something to which one can attribute purpose based on the sole observation of its mechanical functioning. The use of reason is what allows us to become independent of passion and put the latter under instrumental control.

> The new definition of the mastery of reason brings about an internalization of moral sources. When the hegemony of reason comes to be understood as rational control, the power to objectify body, world, and passions, that is, to assume a thoroughly instrumental stance towards them, then the sources of moral strength can no longer be seen as outside of us in the traditional mode....
>
> (Taylor, 1989, pp. 151–152)

According to Lacan, it is Descartes who sets up the premises of the modern subject and the subject of science (Lacan, 1966). Modernity required the Cartesian *cogito* to become "modern" in its fully-fledged form. At the beginning of modern science, the Galilean mathematization of physics was the first step towards desubjectifying phenomena. Individual sensitive qualities, or any property of what subjectivity is, would be of no interest to the subject of science. "The qualitative markers of empirical individuality, whether psychic or somatic, do not apply to this subject" (Milner, 2021, p. 22). Specifically, the subject of science must empty itself of all personal positioning in relation to the phenomenon. At the very least, any hint of one's own judgment from a first-person perspective must be reduced, even annulled, in order to capture the essence of the phenomenon. The *cogito ergo sum* ("I think, therefore I am") indicates that thinking is an act that can be detached from the subject, since doubt permeates that act of thinking. Thinking does not seem to require an author, but it does require someone to appropriate it and claim it as their own. Any thought whatsoever will only lead one to conclude that *I am* because it is *I* who thought. In this, the phenomenon of depersonalization in the psychotic experience is best translated by Modernity, by the Cartesian step that inaugurated the modern and scientific subject as subjects who can be dispossessed and distanced from their own act of thinking, who can take themselves as objects.

> We can then see why Lacan only signs on to what we can call the extreme point of the *cogito*, and why he makes every effort to stop the movement from the first moment to the second. This is why he limits the *cogito* to its enunciation alone, and why he, moreover, loops this enunciation back onto itself, making the conclusion ("therefore, I am") into the pure *pronuntiatum* of the premise ("I think"): "to write: *I think: 'therefore I am'*, with quotation marks around the second clause" ("Science and Truth," Lacan 2006m, 734). This ensures that a thought without qualities persists, ceasing just before it differentiates itself into doubt, conception, affirmation, negation, etc.
>
> (Milner, 2021, p. 23)

Descartes' turn gives rise to the divided subject (*Spaltung*), causing a disjunction in the acts of the modern individual, who is simultaneously in control and out of control of its personal qualities. This division is a product of the chain of signifiers, or a consequence of Language. In Lacanian terms, Language is the structure, and *Spaltung* is the division that the subject feels in the different formations of the unconscious, where something speaks beyond what is spoken. This suggests, without further ado, that psychosis, as psychiatry would describe it a century later (*e.g.*, William Battie or Joseph Daquin), begins to take the place of the most extreme result of Modernity, as Modernity on the edge of the cliff. The psychotic is an open witness to feeling spoken through, alienated by the Other, and experiencing division in its starkest form. As a result, the psychotic requires a type of intervention by the new social regulation entities, such as medicine, justice, prison, etc. Just as the subject of science is a product of Modernity, so too it seems is the "psychotic subject".

For Descartes, scholastic philosophy, theology, magic, or alchemy no longer promoted any strict relationship between what is perceived and thought, as something coming from the will of God; what is perceived and thought does not come from any divine source. The texts of those "sciences" no longer had any clue on how to interpret the occurrences, events, symbols, and facts of the world. Nature would function mechanically, and thus God would have preserved it forever, "thus that there may be many changes in its parts that cannot, it seems to me, properly be attributed to the action of God..." (Descartes, 1998, p. 25). Nature can be studied without having to think about God, totally separated from his will.

8.4. The psychotic, or the Real martyr of Language

From Bacon and Descartes, with the beginning of Modernity in the 16th and 17th centuries, we can jump to Nietzsche, the first to dare to announce what his two predecessors were not capable of: the death of God. Now, this statement, as equivocal and evocative as it may seem, does not indicate that religion is dead, or that the idea of God has disappeared. On the contrary, while God continues to remain "dead" (still unrevealed and now refuted; the end of the suprasensory world) the more the options of faith will multiply. Lacan believes that the image of modern man unveiled a stark contrast to the predictions of late 19th-century thinkers. Modern man appeared both pitiable compared to the utopian visions of libertarians and disturbingly vacuous next to the moralists' anxieties about secularization and social fragmentation (Lacan, 1950).

However, it does indicate that a point in the history of humanity has been reached in which the human ends up discovering his own loneliness, the incompleteness of the Other, its castration. Now, for Lacan, this idea of God as dead is exactly where the Law and the prohibition are grounded. The fact that God is dead confronts us with our own castration and with the abyss of meaning that opens before us. It was Modernity that brought with it the discovery of the death of God and of the father of the Old Testament and of myths. Now, myths like *Enuma Elish* or Freud's primal horde parricide highlight their pivot point in the murder and death of the father or an ascendant, and it's after this that Law and order are mobilized; it requires a paradoxical stance to institute humanity.

The death of God left the Master totally adrift, unable to rely on God to prescribe commandments. Now, the Master has no choice but to turn to himself and his own resources. He must assume himself as an autonomous ego, owner of his actions and destiny. The psychotic subject is one of those who must pay the price of being a master without ties, apparently master of himself, but torn from a signifier that guarantees him a place within the discursive order in which he is immersed.

Now, the neurotic will be no less of a victim of the discourse of Modernity, and is no less disoriented than the psychotic in the universe of discourse. However, as Lacan said, unlike the psychotic, a part being a martyr (etymologically a "witness") of Language the neurotic will be able to find its place in discourse. On the contrary, "the psychotic, in the sense in which he is in a first approach an open witness, seems arrested, immobilized, in a position that leaves him incapable of authentically restoring the sense of what he witnesses and sharing it in the discourse of the others" (Lacan, 1955–1956, p. 132).

In his Seminar *The Sinthome*, after the presentation of a patient at the Hôpital Sainte-Anne, Lacan comments on how this psychotic subject witnessed the way words were imposed upon him.

> That, at least, was how the patient himself articulated something that appears to be all that is most sensible in the realms of an articulation that I may say to be a Lacanian articulation. How is it that any of us can help feeling that the words on which we depend are in some sense imposed upon us?
>
> It is precisely in this respect that he who is called ill sometimes goes further than he who is called a man of sound mind. Rather, the question is why a normal man, a man said to be normal, doesn't notice that speech is a parasite, that speech is a veneer, that speech is a form of cancer that afflicts the human being? How is it that there are some who go so far as to sense this?
>
> (Lacan, 1975–1976, p. 78)

Lacan seems to reverse normality or, at least, question it. He argues that words are a veneer, a coverup, that the normal subject is unaware of and does not experience as imposed, even though they belong to the Other and the subject is alienated by it. For Lacan, the psychotic is closer to the structure of speech in its dependence on a Language that does not belong to it. The psychotic is the true witness and rebel of Language, since he is not willing to live with the Other's words, of which he does not feel the owner, as such. The "normal" person is the one who is striking and questionable because they have to carry out all kinds of intricate procedures so as not to live language and speech as impositions. Modernity would have slackened or even withdrawn the grip of pre-modern Man, questioning the truth of a Language coming from that Other geared to traditions and Catholicism, to the Monarch and the Feudal Order. Now, the psychotic becomes the true representative of Modernity, a man truly free from the chains of Language, as Lacan would say.

We can go on to conclude that the historical observation of cases of psychosis—as described by psychiatry for the past two centuries—really dating from the beginning of Modernity, are largely related to the disappearance of a certain referential power based on myth, of an ordering figure. It is about the transfer of a primordial and structuring signifier within a certain tradition where the acts of speech counted as agents of an organization of subjectivity for individuals. These acts were warranted by the collectivity, sanctioned in principle within the family circle, the closest institutional eventuality. The divorce with the big Other will have to be lived in *sui generis* ways within modern families: some will find a way based on castration and the phallic signifier, although without guarantees; others will have to manage otherwise the incompleteness of the Other.

Where is the family in this change towards Modernism? Where are the Father and Father-God located in this mutation?

Note

1 Before Foucault's (1988) *Madness and Civilization*, there had been no social structuring of the cultural experience of madness. Foucault looked for an answer to the following questions: can the social and collective articulation of madness be described? What are the social fields and institutions behind the treatment and definition of madness? How can the history of knowledge be made, and how do the objects of knowledge arise for a science? There is a subjective pole of the first-person experience of madness and another third-person pole of those who study it. Foucault tries to indicate how insanity and the mentally ill emerge as social constructs. Unlike Littlewood and Dein (2013), Foucault is not concerned with when more cases of schizophrenia appeared in history, but rather with what factors contributed to the moral and political support necessary to apply the term "schizophrenia" or insanity to certain people.

The different ages in the Western world included the construction of categories around power and the way of controlling people, which ended up being normalized. In the Middle Ages, it was the uncontaminated vs. leprosy, life in accordance with values vs. death; in the Renaissance, it was an implied opposition between prudence vs. folly; to stay on the side of prudence, you no longer had to avoid death but madness, beggary, and impurity. Finally, reason and unreason became the twofold borders for a morally sanctioned life in Modernity. The Great Confinement arose as a means to exclude by forcing the mad, the vagabond, the debauched, the unreasonable, etc., to be locked up and employed as a working force in the rising capitalist system.

9

From the conjugal family to the NotF

A look at a misguided conception of the family

9.1. Durkheim's hypothesis of the termination of the extended family and the decline of the father

In his text *Les complexes familiaux dans la formation de l'individu*, Lacan examines the family and its transformation from extended, patriarchal (primitive family), and paternal families (stem family) to the conjugal family, which occurred in the 19th century. Markos Zafiropoulos suggests that Émile Durkheim and Frédéric Le Play, considered the founders of sociology, promulgated the idea of a profound mutation of the family as a consequence of the French Revolution and, later, the rise of the modern state. The latter would have promoted a break with traditional ways of life, leading to the appearance of the reduced family of the conjugal type, anomie, and a decline of the paternal image. Durkheim postulates that the "law of family contraction" promoted not only the reduction of the family institution but also changes in the relationship between its members and in the bond with the family assets. The stem and paternal families of the Old Regime placed the father as the head, as moral and religious authority, the figure of the great Patriarch, who could dominate not only over blood relatives but over a larger group. He made key decisions and decided over their destinies. The group swirled around this personality.

> And, as it thus embodied the entire group, men and things, this personality found itself invested with an authority that placed both things and men under its dependence; thus individual property was born. It was with the advent of paternal power, and more especially patriarchal power, that this transformation took place. We have seen how... it became a high moral and religious power; the whole life of the group is absorbed by it; thus, the leader has the same superiority as the collectivity over each of its members. He was the family being personified.
> (Durkheim, 2000, pp. 387–388 [*Translated by the author*])

According to Zafiropoulos (2002), Durkheim situates the emergence of the reduced, conjugal family in the Germanic tradition, where the paternal family allowed one of their children to become emancipated once married, forming their own life, unlike the Roman family, where married children lived under the same

DOI: 10.4324/9781032663616-12

roof and under the authority of the father. In the Germanic tradition, the couple's assets would belong to them and no longer to the stem family.

The rise of the modern state eventually displaced the figure of the *pater familias*, leading to his downfall. The French Civil Code of the 19th century determined the composition of the family, the decline of the father's jurisdiction, and his role as an authority figure. In Durkheim's words, this led to increased individualism on the one hand, and decreased group solidarity on the other, since there were no longer common goods within an extended circle. From then on, everything depended on the relationship between the immediate marital couple.

> In more general lines, we can say that the decline of the domestic patrimony that would constitute ('since always') the material and sacred foundation of the collective consciousness of the family group is accompanied, in Durkheim's opinion, by the weakening of this consciousness and the appearance of a kind of modern individualism pregnant with moral misery.
>
> (Zafiropoulos, 2002, p. 71 [*Translated by the author*])

All this moral misery would have brought with it consequences such as anomie, individualism, and suicide, according to the sociologist.

9.2. The rebuttal. Lacan's new approach to the decline of the father

This reading of the conjugal family as the result of Modernity was refuted in the 1970s by a succession of works by sociologists and historians who pointed out that the conjugal family predominated in Europe long before the French Revolution, or even Modernity. The conjugal family was the prototype of humble, peasant, or simply uprooted families, the extended or stem family being rather rare or limited to aristocratic circles or great feudal houses. In the Middle Ages, most people, poor or immigrants, did not even know what a lineage was nor even had surnames; they didn't even know what extensive cohabitation meant. They lived either with their partner, in small towns at host sites, or in a disseminated manner. Many even grew up in orphanages without knowing what a family was.

> The economy of marital property predominates among the poor, while that of the rich is combined with that of lineage; in precariousness, it cannot even be constituted. [...] The dominant idea is that the further the investigations go back in time, the more the existence of the couple and their economy are verified at all times and places, even though the history of the family is not reduced... to the extension of the conjugal family.
>
> (Zafiropoulos, 2002, p. 158 [*Translated by the author*])

Lacan would end up detouring from this idea of the law of family contraction, even moving away from Durkheim. For the former, it is no longer a question of an imago of the father, not even of the father person incarnated in any man. In 1953, Lacan gave a conference entitled *The neurotic's individual myth* (*Le mythe individuel du névrosé*), where he used the term "name of the father" for the first time. It is a study and reinterpretation of Freud's case the Rat Man (Freud, 1909a). In this new reading, the structure of the neurosis of the Rat Man, Ernst Lanzer, is articulated in a similar way to the way myths are articulated. Lanzer's story is organized around his Oedipus complex and shows how Lanzer's father, even when dead as while Lanzer was attending Freud, played a Symbolic and Imaginary role in his fantasies and obsessive manifestations, as well as in his own story of life (Lacan, 1953). Lanzer was plagued by obsessive thoughts that always revolved around the idea of his father's death, whether directly at his own hands or indirectly. For Lanzer, the fatherly figure was a major obstacle to his desires. He envisioned his father as an omnipotent and depriving figure. Lacan describes the father not just as an imago, but also as a Symbolic function: a structural element that is distinct from and incompatible with the man who embodies the father role in a family. If Lanzer's father is characterized by something, it is being lacking and flawed. Lacan considers that the flesh-and-blood father allows the binding to a symbolic value, which is in conjunction with a debasement of the person of the father and with the image of the master, the master of moral values, which opens the way for the subject to moral conscience and wisdom (Lacan, 1953). The Father then embodies two seemingly antagonistic readings of the place that this signifier occupies as an empty set. Yet, even as this signifier remains undefined, the parental discourse, right from its inception, starts hinting at the elements that might fall within its scope. Thus, the NotF will be a signifier for a supposed or expected function that operates as a structural function organizing the psyche.

> Thus, from 1953, the power of the father and the structural value of his function no longer obey, for Lacan, so much his social power or that of the group of which he is the head, but rather the value that is proper to him in the Symbolic register. In this perspective, the father of the extended family is not more valuable than the father of the conjugal one. Here the displacement of the social value of the father to the properly symbolic value of his name occurs.
>
> (Zafiropoulos, 2002, pp. 192–193 [*Translated by the author*])

For Lanzer, the Symbolic father can be introduced within a "family romance". This is a kind of lucubration or mythical formation that is similar to the way that little Hans constructed theories about the origin of children and the mystery of the phallus. Lacan argues that the Symbolic father is an ideal that can never be fully embodied by the man who plays the role of the father in a family. This means that each neurotic individual must construct their own meaning based on the ideal of the father (and their identification with the Imaginary father), the place they believe they occupy in the family constellation, and the family myth that they have internalized. This myth is made up of what is said or rumored about them, as well as what is alluded to or between the lines of the comments of their parents, siblings, grandparents, etc. Within his own myth, Lanzer repeats his father's mistakes through identification. He becomes the bearer of his father's debts and decides to marry a rich woman instead of a poor one whom he truly loved, just as his father did.

In Levi-Straussian terms, Lanzer re-enacts the mythemes of the father's historical myth. Lacan provides a structural analysis of Rat Man's case, which can be displayed (Lucchelli, 2010; Gómez Camarena, 2018). The family romance overlaps with his individual myth, meaning that Lanzer inherits the myth of the father as a moral obligation and must figure out how to reconcile this obligation with his own desire. As Lacan reminds us, this is the point where "myth and fantasy reunite" (Lacan, 1953, p. 416), between the family romance and the individual myth (together with his identifications with the Imaginary father).

In contrast to Lanzer, Schreber's father is displaced onto the persecutory figure of God. In addition to being a persecutor, God is also literally an emasculating father. He is a God who demands voluptuousness, limitless jouissance in a feminine form, and at the same time, he is the figure that could provide some appeasement to such disturbing sensations. There is no Symbolic father or NotF that could contain this overwhelming "all" God; the overwhelming jouissance. Schreber searches for something that would stop this desultory experience, bypassing the spiral where he finds himself in the grip of an unbridled jouissance. Lanzer, on the contrary, seems to be looking for something to boost himself, to remove the obstacles from his way. Lanzer appears to be crushed by the ideals of his Imaginary father. He seeks to break free from these moorings by acting clumsily, compulsively, and self-inhibitingly. As a result, he experiences himself as already castrated, meaning that he is impeded in the fulfillment of his desire and cut off from the object of his desire. The Oedipus complex traces an unresolved aspect for Lanzer around his Imaginary father, the father he thought he had, and the Real father, who persists in the background of his actions and significations as an oppressive figure.

Schreber and Lanzer are both children of Modernity in the sense that they must assume their individuality. This means taking ownership of one's duty to become oneself, a mandate that has become personal in the era of individual autonomy. This shift has also generated certain changes in the relationship with the Symbolic father, or NotF.

The Symbolic father no longer seems to hold the same sway in the face of individualizing pressures. The semblance of the Imaginary father now depends on the way the Symbolic father has been inscribed, such that the modern individual can deny, question, or even reject the Imaginary father altogether. However, the Symbolic father persists as a name and surname that is delegated to children, and his rank as a signifier is maintained. Parenting and identifying with a father have become problematic for the modern individual because they have become a choice and a function with a higher responsibility. The Platonic-Augustinian inwardness that progressively expanded in the West, as Taylor suggests, bestows something crucial to the autonomous individual: another form of semblance. It grants the individual the illusion of freedom, but leaves it utterly helpless to ensure the truthfulness of its choices. The Cartesian and Baconian transcendental subject is not master of itself, and there is no transparency to its own will and decision-making.

9.3. A critique on Modernity's illusion: the autonomous ego

Where does the ego-ideal reside, now that it is no longer guaranteed by function or identification with the Imaginary father? In his neurosis, Lanzer can resort to the paternal metaphor and the individual myth, but Schreber must resort to the delusional metaphor and build something out of nothing. Lacan's insights into the modern movement of the death of God and the liberation of Man focus on the ideal of autonomy that Man is pursuing. He argues that this autonomy is an illusion, a semblance, because it is ultimately sustained by a constitutive heteronomy, that is, Man's dependence on the Other and its desire. The subject is alienated by language, not only submitting to it but also being forced to make a choice between being and meaning. This is what I meant by the concept of alienation in Chapter 2. The subject is called a subject precisely because it is subjected to an Other and its signifiers but at the same time must turn into a *modern* subject.

> A certain breathing space is indispensable to modern man, one in which his independence from him not only of any master but also of any god is affirmed, a space for his irreducible autonomy from him as individual, as individual existence. Here there is indeed something that merits a point-by-point comparison with a delusional discourse. It's one itself. It plays a part in the modern's individual presence in the world and in his relations with his counterparts.
>
> (Lacan, 1955–1956, p. 133)

Lacan argues that the discourse of modernity is delusional because the modern subject is caught in a double tension. On the one hand, the subject must conform to the demands of the Other, which is Lacan's term for the Symbolic order of language and culture. This includes the demands of social institutions and norms, as well as the desires of others (our peers). On the other hand, the subject also has its own desires, which may conflict with the demands of the Other. The ego of Modernity is an empty container that is filled with any ideological discourse and a narcissistic tendency overlapping this content. For example, Lanzer lives his speech through an experience that maintains a certainty of the presence of a paternal and phallic signifier that delivers him a truth. This signifier sustains some desire beyond the demands that the subject states or tries to address; there is an Other who does not forsake him and then comes back to squeeze him. However, Lanzer still has to live the dichotomy of his desire and the desire of the Other. On the other hand, Schreber must bear an Other that leaves him trapped in that swing, and when he feels forsaken "different phenomena from those of the continuous internal discourse arise—things slow down, there are interruptions, discontinuities, which the subject is forced to complement. [...] is accompanied by sensations that are very painful for the subject" (Lacan, 1955–1956, pp. 139–140).

The speaking subject is always structurally heteronomous, regardless of its subject-position. This is what Lacan called the operation of alienation, the inclusion of the subject ($) in the set of A. The ideal of full individual autonomy in Modernity is completely exposed when the hypothetical modern individual realizes that its liberty, free choice, and decision-making will always inevitably have to go through the Other and confront it with its own narcissistic tendencies and the desire of the Other. Lacan's aphorism, *man's desire is the desire of the Other*, comes to the forefront here, regardless of whether the genitive is subjective or objective. The psychotic embodies what it means to be a puppet of the Other's desire, whether it is the psychotic's own unknown desire or the desire of the Other that drags it along. Whereas the neurotic is precisely stuck between desiring the Other and desiring the desire belonging to the Other. Even the ascetic anchorite who isolates himself from the community and renounces material objects to dedicate himself to preaching and penance, Freud reminds us in his reply to Jung (Freud, 1915), cannot completely separate himself from the Other; he had to go through a libidinal sublimation for ascetic purposes. That is, the Other remains under a fantasized and imaginary figure, apparently separated from sexual ends, but it continues to be invested libidinously. The neurotic can leave the Other behind, and even may feel forsaken by it, but will maintain a libidinal cathexis of it. Its symptom will swirl around this Other as a continuous source of mystery.

Hence, for the schizophrenic, or even the paranoic, even if they withdraw their libido from objects and the Other, "*[t]he delusional formation, which we take to be a pathological product, is in reality an attempt at recovery, a process of reconstruction*" (Freud, 1911, p. 71). This means that the psychotic seeks as a self-healing and reconstructive need, after the "internal catastrophe", to reconnect with the Other and to cathexe it libidinally through this speech device.

9.4. The triggering of psychosis and the encounter with the One-father

The foregoing can be related to the way in which Lacan describes how the triggering of a psychosis occurs. In *On a question prior...* he points out that it is in the encounter with One-father (*Un-père*), who appears as a symbolic opposition to an Imaginary couple (*a-a'*) needing the NotF to convey such encounter, that psychosis is triggered (Lacan, 1959, p. 481). It is One-father because it already begins to count as one and as a father when it acquires a signifying value in the Symbolic chain, that is, when it is incarnated in something beyond a flesh-and-blood person, thus a paternal function or ideal. However, Lacan points out: "[b]ut how can the Name-of-the-Father be summoned by the subject to the only place from which it could have come into being for him and in which it has never been? By nothing other than a real father... by One-father" (Lacan, 1959, p. 481). The psychotic finds no response to this encounter, staggers, and a collapse of the Imaginary occurs. In the case of Schreber, for example, his psychosis is triggered at first when he is asked to be a member of the Reichstag and a second time when he is appointed president of the Supreme Court. Running into an Imaginary father and its Symbolic status confronts the subject with the Real father, which emerges when he was inclined to respond to a paternal function and ideal: occupying a place of authority and power. Many psychoanalysts will say that this paternal function and ideal would not be the only triggers for psychosis or would not be sufficient; they are necessary but not sufficient. For example, encounters with the desire of the Other or with an inexplicable jouissance are also observed as triggering situations for many psychoses (Redmond, 2014; Vanheule, 2019). However, generally, these onsets imply the peer (small other, peer, or the other in the mirror), or an Imaginary encounter (*a-a'*) with a fellow being, to whom a place is imaginarily attributed and who suggests or sets in motion a certain subjective initiative, proper to an individual, where it is expected that it assumes itself as an *I* (*je*), in a committed speech. Entering the Master's discourse of Modernity, or having to accommodate oneself within this discourse, or producing a committed speech, fizzle in psychotic crisis for many subjects. Being master of oneself, of one's desire and jouissance, appears as a social requirement in Western societies, and the caregivers of the child who enters the language must lead it to appropriate a speech and then assume the logic of such dominant socio-cultural discourse. Throughout this process, in those first encounters with the mother or maternal caregiver, as I showed in Chapter 5, something of interest is at stake in the inscription of the signifier NotF, which necessarily implies the intervention of speech and the commitment of the Other. If this does not happen, the subject will be disarmed with respect to this Symbolic and discursive assumption, and it will run straight into the Real of the position of a modern Master. This is, faced with the Other's malevolence or the Other as an enjoyer.

In the third part of the book, I will show how a social ontology of discourse can favor a different understanding and approach to psychosis. The passage through an author like J. Searle, and his contribution to status function declarations and speech, acts for an event to count as an event. The legitimacy of an event as an institutional fact presupposes not only a common agreement or a collective recognition but also that the Language and structure arrange the forms in which we deal with desire, jouissance, and actions. How is psychosis inserted within this logic?

10

Depicting the Father in Modernity and Postmodernity

The theatre of Claudel and the cinema of the Coen brothers

> The father would have not to be only the *name-of-the-father*, but also the representative, in all its fullness, of the symbolic value crystallized in his function. Now, it is clear that this coincidence of the symbolic and the real is totally elusive. At least in a social structure like ours, the father is always in one way or another in disharmony with regard to his function, a deficient father, a *humiliated* father, as Claudel would say.
>
> (Lacan, 1953, p. 423)
>
> Lacan, J. (1953). "The neurotic's individual myth". *The Psychoanalytic Quarterly*, 48(3): 405–425, 1979. Reprinted by permission of Taylor & Francis Ltd, http://www.tandfonline.com.

10.1. The father between Modernity and Postmodernity

The epigraph ends with a reference to a well-known author in traditional literary and dramatic circles, coinciding with the first appearance of the NotF concept in Lacan's work. This is no coincidence. Paul Claudel, a poet, diplomat, and playwright of the late 19th and early 20th centuries, was considered the writer of Catholicism. His works permeate questions about religion and faith; the Father, God the Father, and their earthly representatives are present themes in his theater and writings, along with the conception of religious conviction and the conversion of non-believers. The literature and art of an era reflect the subjective coordinates of the epoch, but they also allow for the full performative and exemplary use of psychoanalytic concepts to be displayed wherever speech is used and desire and jouissance operate.

As B. Fink (2004) indicates, in his work, Lacan tends to be more declarative than demonstrative, using performative rather than demonstrative acts to prove his point through the employment of examples. The journey across *Hamlet* and *Antigone* in the Seminars *Desire and Its Interpretation* and *The Ethics of Psychoanalysis*, respectively, show how important theatrical dramas are to Lacan when he looks at how psychoanalysis and its concepts are used in concrete situations and representations. Literary narratives have the same value as unconscious formations and myths because they favor the interpretive production of latent thoughts and

DOI: 10.4324/9781032663616-13

unpresented content. Myths help with structuring the subjectivity of an epoch more than they are constituted by it. Thus, Lacan states:

> For, in short, what are the great mythical themes that creative poems have been testing their mettle against throughout the ages? This long series of variations for centuries upon centuries is nothing but a sort of long approximation that is such that the myth, whose every possibility has been exploited, ends up by entering, strictly speaking, into our subjectivity and psychology. I maintain, and I will unambiguously maintain—and in doing so I believe that I am following in Freud's footsteps—that poetic creations generate psychological creation more than they reflect them.
>
> (Lacan, 1958–1959, p. 248)

Psychoanalysis offers a new way of understanding the socio-political context, the drama, and the performance of the unconscious and desire in human relationships. Individuals are shaped not only by their families, but also by larger myths and tragedies. These tragedies reflect the structure of the subjectivity of a particular context, but also help shaping it. In this case, it is important to understand the role of the Father in one of the critical moments of Modernity, before authors such as Jean-François Lyotard, Gianni Vattimo, and Gilles Lipovetsky declared the end or definitive transformation of Modernity. This transformation includes the end of grand, overarching narratives of reality. Now, there are many metanarratives, and each individual or community can create their own. Lyotard defines metanarratives as theories or discourses that seek to provide an overarching, comprehensive, and legitimizing explanation of both major social events and diverse cultural phenomena, assuming a universal or objective truth (Lyotard, 1984). The great metanarratives of Modernity—the Enlightenment, science, capitalism, and Marxism—failed, demonstrating their fallibility and disappointing 20th and 21st-century citizens. This initiated a period of transformation of Modernity that Lyotard calls Postmodernity.

Lipovetsky, on the other hand, speaks of hypermodernity and the "age of emptiness" as the core of Modernity itself. In this hypermodern era, hyper-individualism leads to an uprooting of historical context and narratives, and hedonism and narcissistic tendencies take priority. The main objective is the total fulfillment of the personal ego, but an ego disconnected from the other. Truth relativism predominates, and there is a substantial disengagement of the individual from the *res publica* (Lipovetsky, 2000).

Where does the Father stand at the beginning of this fracture? Claudel's theater seems to illustrate what happens to the Father in Modernity, on the eve of its transformation. Claudel said that "faith makes every modern man live in an essentially dramatic environment". Do Postmodernity and hypermodernity propose a mutation of the Father's place? Perhaps the cinema of recent years can shed light on the role of the father in Postmodernity. The work of the Coen brothers can serve as a reference, especially their three films that could be considered the "trilogy of the father": *Fargo, No Country for Old Men,* and *A Serious Man*. The film *Raising Arizona* should probably be included in this anthology but due to its comedic character and in order to maintain the trilogical aspect of the parallel with Claudel I will not analyze it. However, this film, more than any of the others, explicitly poses the question of being a father in Postmodernity. A fact that perhaps the cinephile reader won't hesitate to rebuke.

Before we proceed, what exactly is it about the father that is exposed, degraded, or affected in Modernity and Postmodernity? Is it the flesh-and-blood person who embodies him that appears humiliated and scorned? I could answer that the issue is not so much about the individual who occupies that place, nor even the tasks or functions of a father, or the characteristics that the Other attributes to him, such as "thundering father, easy-going father, all-powerful father, humiliated father, rigid father, pathetic father, stay-at-home father, [or] father on the loose" (Lacan, 1959, p. 482). Lacan calls the Symbolic father the floating signifier of the Law and the first body of the signifier. As long as someone enacts this rank and status, promotes it in their speech and actions, and shows a degree of commitment to sustaining and living it, the signifier of the Father will persist and be engaged, even if the NotF is spreading and the Father is made to survive in new ways. Even though the person of the father is "the people who makes the laws or presents himself as a pillar of faith, as a paragon of integrity or devotion, as virtuous or a virtuoso...as serving the nation or the birth rate... legacy or law... or the empire" (Lacan, 1959, p. 482), the child will be able to see through it his hypocrisy, his flaws, and what is in contradiction with what that signifier should represent and stand for in the realm of the Law. This is even less so if the companion, be it the mother or whoever takes her place, does not legitimize and validate the actions, the speech, and the entire signifying framework of the father's person when he conveys or seeks to put that NotF signifier into play.

If something is humiliated, it is not so much the character or the person as the paternal signifier, where what is expected of that signifier in the human world is distorted. Now, some Lacanian circles have sought to appeal to the father and denounce his disappearance, even suggesting the "return of the matriarchy" and a "society of fundamentally homosexual masters" (Melman, 2009). However, these claims are questionable and somewhat exaggerated. The role of the father is not in peril, nor is the person who embodies the father being relegated. He is not losing his masculinity or his power as a father in a society that is supposedly becoming feminized and returning to matriarchy, something that has never existed in history. The father, as the signifier NotF in the Other {A}, is not fully inscribed or assumed in its purely Symbolic value. In other words, no one can totally and completely monopolize or represent the paternal signifier. The problem is both the degradation and aggrandizement of this signifier. Praising it or rejecting it to excess can be harmful, as both can lead to situations that threaten the stability of the social bond.

10.2. The father through the lens of narrative art: the theatre of Paul Claudel and the trilogy of the Coûfontaine

In the epigraph, Lacan refers to Claudel's third drama, *The Humiliation of the Father* (*Le père humilié*), part of the "trilogy of the Coûfontaine". Lacan devotes a section of his Seminar *Transference* to commenting on this trilogy, which also includes the previous plays *The Hostage* (*L'otage*) and *Crusts* (*Le pain dur*). Lacan calls the trilogy a "modern tragedy, by which I mean that it is contemporary" (Lacan, 1960–1961, p. 271). The story of three generations of the Coûfontaine family unfolds during the first half of the 19th century, a century of revolutionary change. The Coûfontaine family, an aristocratic dynasty, pays the price for the French Revolution, losing their lands and legacy. The plots of the plays swirl around this family's struggles, set against the backdrop of a rapidly changing world. This is a very specific period of Modernity, marked by the birth of the bureaucratic-democratic state, secularism, the separation of powers, political constitutions, the Industrial Revolution, and the consolidation of capitalism and individualism in Europe and the West. It is also a time when Marxism emerges.

In the first play, *The Hostage*, Sygne de Coûfontaine wants to recover the family name and lands, her father's legacy. She is willing to marry her cousin to save that family name along with the land, but she betrays all this by marrying the family enemy, usurper, and son of a sorcerer, baron and prefect Toussaint Turelure. She sacrifices herself to save her cousin and the pope from the menaces Turelure casts on the former. The pope lodges undercover in her domain and could be in danger if found by Turelure.

In the second play, *Crusts*, Louis de Coûfontaine, the son of Sygne and Turelure, in collusion with his father's mistress, Sichel, and a usurer and lover of Louis, Lumîr, who is demanding repayment of a loan agreed so as to save some of Louis' lands in Algeria, decides to assassinate his father. A man depicting the begetter of the primal horde, killed for the value of the property that the usurer and his son demanded of him (Sauret, 2009).

Finally, the third drama involves Pensée, the blind daughter of Louis and Sichel, who is in love with Orian, the pope's nephew, and Orso's brother. She becomes pregnant by him, but they won't remain together because the pope convinces him to leave her since he is a true catholic and she is a Jew; he later goes to war where he dies. She then marries Orso without loving him, indeed their union is only in order to give her child a father.

According to Lacan, the phantom of the "humiliated father" haunts the three oeuvres of the trilogy; it happens to be either an embodied character or subtextual idea. He is not only incarnated in the figure of the pope, who appears twice in the first and third dramas. For Lacan, the key and central character of the father and the representative of the degradation of its Symbolic status and signifier is Toussaint Turelure, who appears in the first but especially in the second play as the father murdered by the son, the prototype of the Real-primordial father and of the Oedipus tragedy.

> The father whose stature verges on a kind of obscenity, the father whose stature is strictly speaking impudent, the father in whom we cannot fail to note certain echoes of the ape-like form in which Freud's myth [of the primal horde] makes him appear at the horizon.
>
> (Lacan, 1960–1961, p. 284)

The father becomes the object of derision and contempt, bordering on the abject. In *Crusts*, the character of Turelure, now aged and diminished, is a father whose only concerns are his material possessions and his Symbolic position as patriarch. He is therefore interchangeable and always replaceable. He is not willing to give his son the part of the money that both he and his mistress are demanding, nor is he willing to let him succeed him as patriarch. Furthermore, Turelure suspects from the beginning of the play that his son wants him dead, even that he wants to kill him, foreshadowing the play's conclusion. This death, however, does not occur before him trying to usurp his son's fiancée, Lumîr, and take her as his own wife. Dispossessing and stealing from others is how Turelure amassed his wealth and status. During the Reign of Terror, he participated in the execution of the parents and seizure of the assets of Sygne de Coûfontaine's family.

Now, he appears as the figure of the decadent father, the father who causes his humiliation in contrast to the character of the pope, the one who embodies greatness and respect, or, on the other hand, the *pater familias* who delegates the surname Coûfontaine and the lands in *The Hostage*.

> In the tragedy, the pope owes the maintenance of his semblances no longer to God, but to the whim of one of the worst representatives of the *power* of the Empire and to the denial, by a woman, of what founds her bond… in the name and in the father. Claudel allows his reader to wonder about the consequences of this denial for this woman, for the social bond she inhabits, and, above all, for the two generations that follow her… and ultimately, for our time.
>
> (Sauret, 2009, p. 142 [*Translated by the author*])

In *The Hostage*, it was his wife, Sygne, who disavowed Turelure. Now, in *Crusts*, his own mistress, Sichel, detests him, calling him a sinister, nitwitted oldster. She has no qualms about conspiring against him, even urging Louis to kill him. These three plays outline a figure of the woman that opens the way to the changing place of femininity in the social upheavals to come. Lacan notes the prevalence of a castrating mother—more castrating, even, than a father could be. In some way, the female protagonists of Claudel's three dramas represent a woman who questions the father. If castration occurs, it is that of a father who, due to his own inability, lack of desire assumption, and disregard for the women's desire, falls into disgrace with women whose desire is outlined in a mysterious beyond. Does this represent a step towards ~~Woman~~, the Real mother, as a new figure and agent of castration? A surge of the matriarchate? They are complex questions, but they hint in the background at controversial answers that ignite and fuel the debate on the patriarchalism, machismo, and misogyny of which psychoanalysis has been accused.

Does the loss of the father's place and its greater occupation by the mother as a castrating function lead to an increase in psychosis and social turmoil? I don't believe so. First, there has never truly been a matriarchal civilization in human history (Lerner, 1986), so imagining a return to one we know nothing of is dubious. Second, if castration operates, it means that the signifier NotF is functioning to some extent, regardless of who mediates it. The Real father is more a logical operator than some incarnation. Therefore, it is difficult to claim that the throb of the mother as a new castration agent leads to an increase in psychosis and social turmoil.

> The path to which I am trying to redirect you, with the assistance of Claudel's plays, involves re-situating castration at the heart of the problem [of transference]. For castration is identical to what I call the constitution of the desiring subject as such... As I have sufficiently emphasized... castration is identical to the phenomenon that is such that the object that desire lacks—since desire is [based on] lack—is in our experience identical to the very instrument of desire: the phallus.
>
> (Lacan, 1960–1961, pp. 294–295)

The phallus represents that which the subject believes it has or is for the Other. As a signifying function, the phallus helps the subject occupy a place where it can assimilate lack, do something with it, and name and give meaning to it. Above all, this comes down to providing the subject with the signifying means and resources to live with its own lack, the impossibility of the sexual relationship, and the dearth of metalanguage.

10.3. The Postmodern father, the American Dream, and the Coen brothers

How can we illustrate the decline of the father in contemporary narrative works, especially in cinema, which has had a significant impact on popular culture over the past century? Among the metanarratives that rose and fell during this time, the American Dream, or the myth of an enviable nation, was perhaps the most widely-disseminated ideology through art, especially cinema. The American Dream, a metanarrative that has prevailed in cinema and pop culture throughout the 20th and 21st centuries, encompasses the idea of becoming anyone one wishes in a land of opportunity. In order to achieve this dream, one must embrace American values and ways of life, including family, work, wealth, obedience to the law, and unconditional patriotism, even for government enterprises that are warmongering. All of this is done in pursuit of happiness and self-fulfillment. This last term is important because in Postmodernity it means that individuals are less likely to assert social goals than those for personal and individualistic purposes that do not necessarily entail their engagement and sense of duty.

Where does the father fit into this metanarrative? The Founding Fathers and various political and cultural figures in American history may have embodied paternal ego-ideals for many generations, but art and literature have largely been responsible for deconstructing the metanarratives of the father in the context of the American Dream. Despite his multiple depictions, the father retains his character. However, as an agent of castration and a signifier, the father has lost his effectiveness and ability to act, so does this mean that there is an increase in psychotic and borderline traits and transgressions? Does the increase in social disruption, crime, or inequality have, among others, something to do with this decline? On the other hand, and in the opposite direction, does a radical call to a father, its aggrandizement, also mean an increase in political and religious extremism? The U.S. appears to be the country with the most violent deaths by firearms; massacres in schools among children and young students are very frequently making the headlines; the opioid crisis; political and religious extremism; hyper-consumerism and the hyper-concentration of wealth—together with the disappearance of the middle class, these all contribute to cover up the decadence or, its opposite, the infatuation of the father and the meagerness of the metanarrative semblance of the "American Dream".

Joel and Ethan Coen's films have been at the forefront of this process. In movies like *Fargo*, they depict humiliated fathers, blinded by ambition and willing to betray their own families, as in the case of Jerry Lundegaard (William Macy). Jerry is a frustrated middle-class car salesman with ambition who resorts to any means necessary to get money, including hiring two thugs to kidnap his own wife and demand a million-dollar ransom from his father-in-law. Thwarted in his position and further scorned by his father-in-law, Jerry epitomizes the humiliated father. He is the epitome of a small, manipulative, and dishonest man. Aside from his son and wife, of whom we know little, he is the father who best exemplifies impotence, ineptitude, and grotesque behavior. He shatters every ideal of the American Dream when the dream becomes nothing more than an end in itself and others are reduced to mere means to that end. All that remains of a disgraced and poignant father is tragedy. Yet humiliation is not solely produced by the Other; characters like Jerry, with their blinded actions, inflict this humiliation and degradation of the paternal signifier upon themselves. Lacan seems to suggest that humiliation is not always inflicted by unjust Others. Rather, those who embody the paternal signifier may choose to undermine its symbolic, deontic, and apophantic weight. In stark contrast to Jerry Lundegaard, Marge Gunderson (Frances McDormand), the police officer who investigates the crimes related to the kidnapping, embodies certain master signifiers that are fading into secondary status in Postmodernity, such as simplicity, integrity, and moral rectitude.

In *No Country for Old Men*, the three sheriff characters—Ed Bell (Tommy Lee Jones), El Paso sheriff (Rodger Boyce), and retired sheriff Ellis (Barry Corbin)—face a similar predicament. In a changing and degraded world that they no longer understand, they accept their place, even though they are nothing more than forgotten relics of an illusory ideal in a country that no longer belongs to old men. Ed Bell recalls the oldtimers, legends of the law who preceded him, embodying an ideal of law enforcement that he evokes with respect and pride, remembering their exploits and teachings. The film exudes a certain nostalgia and reverence for the Imaginary figure of the father. Ed's calls to the different sheriff figures at the beginning and end of the movie, as well as his dream of his deceased father showing him where he will be waiting for him, are essentially calls to a dead father, one who was never truly there and could not have prevented the debacle or abjection of the world they fought against. Yet these calls reveal a neurotic attachment to and legitimization of the Father as the locus of the signifier S_1, the starting point and referent of the different representations of an ideal metanarrative that, though spurious, still provides meaning, consistency, and order to the world.

The foregoing stands in contrast with the misguided and lawless character who represents the antithesis of the idealized father, or rather the punishing father in the film, Anton Chigurh (Javier Bardem). The pinnacle of the hypermodern man and nemesis of the lawmen, condensed in this character with psychopathic traits, he is the true representative of the foreclosure of the NotF or the return of a primal father. Driven by a full conviction in getting his job done, he has no regard for others and will kill whoever stands in his way, but not before giving them some sort of chance of staying alive in a coin toss.

It is clear that it is not greed that drives Chigurh, but like Eichmann, the responsibility of a job well done that must be fulfilled to its ultimate consequences without minding any ethical considerations that would hinder its correct execution. Chigurh is an excellent employee; he also dispatches and chooses who should be "fired" for incompetence, discarding them with a compressed-air bolt pistol usually employed for cattle sacrificing. He typifies the laws of nature, a sort of *père fouettard* or punitive father, but also the grim reaper. In this, his evil is not banal but fully psychopathic and individualistic, following a solipsistic logic that underpins a Kantian imperative in making the decision of who lives and who dies. All this is more visible in the book on which the film is based than in the film. His modus operandi is so confusing and twisted that even the characters of the drug cartel fear him, and remain bewildered by his actions. So Chigurh represents this ambiguity of the father, either by his total disregard of the law and life, or by generating his own twisted law system that he abides by. So, in this, he is a total self-made individual, with a different moral code, who epitomizes a sort of judge and executioner that has both demoted and radicalized the father figure.

However, it is perhaps the character of Larry Gopnik (Michael Stuhlbarg) in the film *A Serious Man* that is the most ambiguous and difficult to grasp as a father figure in the Coen brothers' universe. He is a banal character anchored in Modernity, defying stereotypical father figures. He is neither tyrannical and humiliating nor an ego-ideal and representative of the law. He may be closest to Jerry Lundegaard in their naiveté, but without the same degree of paternal debasement. Larry is portrayed as a good citizen, dutiful at home and at work, with a house in the suburbs, a stable job as a university professor, a wife, and two children. He is a serious man who lives the American Dream in full expression. However, things coincidentally start going wrong for him: his wife asks him for a divorce without him understanding why, and she doesn't give him any further explanations; a student tries to bribe him to change his grades; he finds out his neighbor is illegally annexing part of his yard; then his wife tells him to leave the house to give room for her new lover; he meets the lover who later accidentally dies and for whom he must pay for his funeral; then his brother is arrested for solicitation and he must also pay for that; he sees his tenure affected after some anonymous letters are sent to the university speaking ill of him; he sees how his lawyer dies suddenly; he is involved in a car accident; he must pay for a record subscription he never asked for, etc. All this happens to him despite him, even though he insists that "*he didn't do anything*". These calamities push him to search for an answer, but instead of reacting to them, his passivity moves him to embark on an intricate quest for an answer to the mystery of this chain of events. How come after being a good father, a good American citizen, and a serious man who has "*done nothing*", is it possible that everything is turning on its head for him? Why would God have decided to punish him like this? Existential questions encroach on Larry, but there is no interpretation at hand, so he turns to religion for solace. Being a practicing Jew, he meets a junior rabbi who tells him that everything that has happened to him is a matter of perspective, of how we see things—an explanation that fails to convince him. Immediately, he turns to another more experienced rabbi, who answers him with a kind of parable: a Jewish dentist discovered a message in Hebrew ("help me") engraved on the back of the teeth of one of his patients and believing that it was a message from God addressed to him, he incessantly sought to give it meaning and purpose even though it did not have any. However, the parable ends up being just as perplexing as Larry was expecting some sort of closure, something that would offer him a resolution. Finally, he tries to meet with the eldest and wiser rabbi, Marshak, who just doesn't have the time to talk to him, metaphorizing the divine silence before the big questions. Neither religion, culture, nor circumstances can offer Larry any answers; everything just leads to more confusion.

In general, each character in the film seeks to find meaning in life the best they can; his brother elaborates the "mentaculus", some sort of convoluted schizography of the universe; his son and his neighbor smoke weed; and Larry applies tangled mathematical formulae that seek to demonstrate the uncertainty principle and Schrödinger's cat dilemma (which prove that we can never really know "*what's going on*"). None of these explanations can answer the mystery of why things happen to us. The moral lesson resides in the Book of Job, we must endure the mishaps of life and accept destiny, as Job says to God after his trials: "Therefore I have uttered what I did not understand, things too wonderful for me, which I knew not" (King James Bible, Job 42: 3). The big existential questions about human life and purpose turn out to be overwhelmingly simple, and they remind the modern and postmodern subject that there is no big Other of certainty and with prefabricated answers to all its conundrums.

Not only as a modern individual is Larry questioned, but also his place as a father and a husband, since he is not taken seriously by his wife or his children in a marriage that collapses without him even knowing why. Larry is the paradigm of a man of inaction and total passivity who, in his parsimony, accepts everything that happens to him without much response, supposing that for his good deeds, fate should reward him. Tragedy or bad news need not knock on his door if he has minimized the risks by acting under the ethical premises of Judaism. However, his total position of naivete and passivity make him look like a character without desire, without initiative, lacking decision, and what happens to him is not simply a matter of fate or God playing tricks on him. It is precisely not fully assuming the lack and the phallic signifier, neither as a father, a husband, or an employee, that leads to what he did not expect to happen to him.

It is after a dream in which he says goodbye to his brother, who is leaving by boat to start a new life in Canada and is suddenly killed by anti-Semitic hunters, that Larry begins to restore the life he previously had. The Symbolic death of the older brother, a depleted and faded father figure, and the bar mitzvah of his son, mark a moment of rupture where the myth of Oedipus and the rite of passage yield to a place for lack. As for Louis de Coûfontaine in *Crusts*, we can say of Larry that "from now on he is no longer going to be a good-for-nothing who botches up everything and who allows his land to be stolen from him... He becomes the father" (Lacan, 1960–1961, p. 323).

10.4. The "father trilogy" as a Postmodern myth

The Coen brothers' "father trilogy" can be seen as a modern myth, responding to Lévi-Strauss' formula for the structure of myth (1963):

$$F_x(a): F_y(b) \approx F_x(b): F_{a-1}(y)$$

This formula can be read as two terms *a* and *b*, and two functions of those terms, F_x and F_y, where $F_x(a)$ conflicts with $F_y(b)$ just as $F_x(b)$ conflicts with $F_{a-1}(y)$. The myth indicates a "twisting" of these relationships and terms "under two conditions: (I) that one term be replaced by its opposite (in the above formula *a* and *a-1*); (2) that an inversion be made between the function value and the term value of two elements (above *y* and *a*)" (Lévi-Strauss, 1963, p. 228). The myth drawn between the three films points to the father's place in the American Dream's meta-narrative and how each of its representatives fits into a role in the achievement of the dream and the conflict that is generated with that dream. The first two films trace the antagonism of the myth, the left side of the formula, where the lawmen, Marge and Ed (*a*), in addition to representing the function of the law, represent the function of the ideal father; the family's and the community's tragic hero, a basis for the Symbolic Father and the ideal of the Father (F_x). Meanwhile, Jerry and Chigurh (*b*) are both the decadent and the punishing father of the primal horde, the antithesis of the "good" and the Symbolic Father (F_y). In *A Serious Man*, representing, in this case, the right side of the formula, the myth assumes the conflict between "good" and "evil" in another way, where the role of the "good" and ideal father is not any representative of the law, as such, but neither is he a truly admirable figure, not even idealizable, like those new figures of the modern hero that cinema seeks to personify in the role of the police officer. Larry is nothing more than a *b* who meets F_x, an ordinary man, a "man in the street" marked by pathos and ridicule. However, here the important question is, who is $F_{a-1}(y)$, the double inversion of the relation and the term? That which favors the closure of the myth—if such can be considered a closure—is something that is outlined in *No Country for Old Men*, but that is not fully evident until *A Serious Man*. The $F_{a-1}(y)$ is nothing more than the hazards of destiny, the flip-flops of time and space, the uncertainty. In this, that function and element, at the same time, are neither "good" or "bad". They are totally purposeless and unintentional. The Coen brothers' myth leaves $F_{a-1}(y)$ as an "irreducible residue", of which Lacan speaks of in his conversation with Lévi-Strauss and other intellectuals about the myth, where he indicates that this residue

> imposes itself as correlative to the transformation of the group: where can be read, what I will say, the sign of a kind of impossibility of the total resolution of the problem of the myth. So that the myth would be there to show us the equation in a signifying form of a problem which must by itself necessarily leave something unanswered, which responds to the insoluble by signifying insolubility and its prominence found in its equivalences, which provides (this would be the function of the myth) the signifier of the impossible.
>
> (Lacan et al., 1956, p. 714 [*Translated by the author*])

The Coen brothers' myth does not leave much room for conflictive resolution between antagonisms; on the contrary, it places antagonism as an impasse without a definitive resolution, although with momentary appeasements, but where contingencies and chance "decide" the succession of events. Precisely, the Coen brothers show that there is no invisible hand behind the events, that there is no divine will pulling the strings, that there is no predestination of lives or incarnate demon seeking evil; behind the amorphous mass of coincidences and adversities, there is no hidden meaning; we are just the random fruit of a universe that does not care about us.

Part 3

A socio-ontological appraisal of psychosis

11

Declarations and discourse, or the intervention of Language in the founding of eventfulness and the subject-position

11.1. What counts as a social fact? The formalization of the social fact in Searle's social ontology

Human society and all the acts that we can classify as "social", or social facts, are based on a principle, an "underlying commonality". In his work on social ontology, John Searle indicates that "status function declarations" (SFD) are the ability to impose functions on objects, people, and situations that could not perform those functions just because of their intrinsic physical structure.

SFDs are performative utterances or speech acts that attribute a social weight to an object, situation, or signifier. John Searle proposed SFDs to describe how social events occur and are sanctioned. He argued that language can make something count as a function if there is a shared understanding of that function. Only then can that thing fulfill its intended purpose. Also, however, some deontic powers have to be mobilized, "that is, they carry out rights, duties, obligations, requirements, permissions, authorizations, entitlements, and so on. [...] [T]hey provide us with reasons for acting that are independent of our inclinations or desires" (Searle, 2010, pp. 8–9). On this last point, Searle's statement may be questionable, as we saw in Chapter 7, desire and Law are closely related and are mutually dependent. This means that any deontic position is entailed by a conative one, or a position of desire.

This philosopher also observes the need for a multiple to start counting-as-one. Based on declarations, or Austin's performative utterances—when we do things with words or when our declarations have effects in the world—we allow a fuzzy multiple to enter the count. Like when the priest sentences at the end of the wedding: "I declare you husband and wife", or when the master exclaims "I hereby order...!", or when the repentant lover says, "I promise...", all are performative speech acts. Dispersed elements of the world or other sets, such as {A}, are taken to generate meaning and truth under a declarative form.

The institutional reality would be given by SFD of this type. So, Searle proposes a formula that summarizes the basic structure of SFD: "X counts as Y in C", C being the context. This author introduces the logic of sets, perhaps without realizing it, in order to describe how an institutional fact is established. Starting from

DOI: 10.4324/9781032663616-15

this minimal structure: "We make it the case by Declaration that X has the status Y and thus is able to perform the function F in C", or, in more detail, Declaration: $\forall_x p(c) \forall_C [x \in Y \leftrightarrow x \in F \leftrightarrow x \in p(c)]$, which can be read as "We make it the case by Declaration that for any x that satisfies the properties of c in any C context, such as x has the status of Y, iff it has the status of function F, and iff x satisfies the conditions of properties c".

Searle sketches the minimum logical structure necessary for an institutional fact. This also implies something that he does not contemplate and is the possibility that there was previously an eventful site (*site événementiel*). According to Badiou, this means an ab-normal multiple for which none of its elements are present in the situation; the site is present but the elements that compose it are "underneath" it, masked. Badiou explains that the eventful site is on the edge of the void and is foundational. Being on the edge of the void means that this type of multiple is made out of unpresented members; none of its terms is counted-as-one because they are close to emptiness. "A site is therefore the *minimal* effect of structure which can be conceived; it is such that it belongs to the situation, whilst what belongs to it in turn does not. [...] Within the situation, this multiple is, but *that of which* it is multiple is not" (Badiou, 2005, p. 175). It is foundational because the multiple is the minimal form for a count to take place. The site allows the count without itself being preceded by any previous one; it is the "first-one" of the situation, thus founding it. For an eventful site to count as an event, it must be related to a historical situation where the events at site X form a multiple, such that its composition includes elements belonging to the site and to itself. Badiou uses the example of the situations that occurred in France between 1789 and 1790, where the series of happenings and riots all over the country constituted the eventful site of something that can be called "The Revolution". Within history, "The Revolution" is the designation that counts as a member of the set.

Badiou tries to distinguish the eventful site from the natural multiplicity. A natural multiplicity is normal by maintaining its qualities as a constant no matter where it presents itself. "Nature is absolute, historicity relative. [...] A multiple is a site relative to the situation in which it is presented (counted-as-one). A multiple is a site solely *in situ*" (Badiou, 2005, p. 176). In contrast, a natural situation is intrinsically definable, preserving its character. Thus, an eventful site is defined locally, whereas a natural situation is global and constant in its qualities. For the eventful site to start counting as an event itself, it must be related to a historicizable situation, where an event of site X is a multiple such as its composition is part of the elements belonging to the site and to itself. Badiou uses this notation:

$$e_x = \{x \in X, e_x\}$$

Where e stands for the event, as a multiple-one of the elements that belong to its site, on the one hand, and to itself, on the other. Where lower case x is or condenses the unpresented element(s) of the eventful site, on the edge of the void. In this sense, Searle's "X counts as Y in C" indicates that C is not just anything, that it is a C loaded with history and possibilities of historicization; composed of presented and unpresented elements. C can count as one or a series of historical events. For C to be the eventfulness of a multiple, a naming and interpretive intervention must be performed. This intervention means "any procedure by which a multiple is recognized as an event" and it consists in "identifying that there has been some undecidability, and in deciding its belonging to the situation" (Badiou, 2005, p. 202). The signifier that is going to compose the designation x is paradoxical because it is not known whether it includes itself. We can then call this first signifier, which initiates the series, S_1. However, that S_1 by itself does not tell us anything if it is not connected in the series with the signified $\{S_1, S_2\}$ or $\{S_2\}$. Hence, there must be *two* for there to be an event, both composed of hidden, unpresented elements, and of a supernumerary name. S_1 names but the name enters the field of interpreted events, as historical, through its link with $\{S_2\}$. Lacan calls that set S_1 "master-signifier"[1], in relation to Hegel's dialectics of the master and the slave, and he calls set S_2 "knowledge". This is knowledge not in the sense of *connaissance* or the way the subject of science relates to the object of its research and the production of an independent/objective knowing, but as *savoir* or the meaning of the articulation of signifiers producing a self-made, truthful knowing about the subject's confrontation with the Real. The master-signifier (S_1) is a position that is embodied and whose function is "to represent the subject for another signifier... However, the subject it represents is not univocal" (Lacan, 1969–1970, p. 89). That S_1 figures as a functional place of operation within discourse. Thus, the discourse shapes the meanings of the actions and the way in which the subject is situated with respect to truth, the Other, knowledge, and jouissance within a sociocultural context. The discourse, for Lacan, is structuring, or it attributes structure. We could situate the NotF as an institutional signifier of discourse that opens the way for the subject. In the meantime, the discourse acts as a support and producer of meaning for linguistic beings.

11.2. From "X counts as Y in C" to Lacan's discourses and the social bond

So far, we have S_1, S_2 and \$ (the lacking or divided subject), three elements that we can count on in the formation of discursive sets. "X counts as Y in C" can be rearranged in another way, and that was what Lacan did in the late 1960s when he proposed his theory of discourses. The concept of discourse in Lacan acquires a relevant meaning for what he intends to propose. First, discourse must be understood as different from speech (*parole*), since discourse supposes a structure of speech and speaking that is configured according to how the agent (desire), the truth, the other, and production (loss) are accommodated within the practices of a social bond. In this, Lacan's proposal differs from that of his contemporaries, M. Foucault or R. Barthes, for whom discourse is a concept with a different intonation and scope. For him, discourse is a *logical formalization* of the way people bond, not through sense or meaning but through the internal relationships between terms and positions that constitute that logic. Therefore, the context and the way the master-signifier, knowledge, the *plus-de-jouir* (the object cause of desire), and the divided subject interact are determined by a preestablished order.

In his later Seminar *Le savoir du psychanalyste*, Lacan proposed four new labels for the four positions of his discourse theory: semblance instead of agent/desire; jouissance instead of the other; and *plus-de-jouir* instead of product/loss (Lacan, 1971–1972a). Discourse is thus seen as a structural and formalized fact that favors the normalization of desire and jouissance. It frames the possible ways in which the social bond is inscribed, but it also depends on that social bond. Lacan even suggests that discourse is "wordless"; it does not require utterances or enunciations.

> The fact is that, in truth, discourse can clearly subsist without words. It subsists in certain fundamental relations which would literally not be able to be maintained without language. [...] There is no need of [enunciations] for our conduct, possibly for our acts, to be inscribed within the framework of certain primordial statements.
>
> (Lacan, 1969–1970, p. 13)

Discourse is basic and pre-verbal, determining the use of words and speech. Our actions and behaviors seem to be grounded in discourse, since it is not just by speaking that we know that someone is engaged in discourse. In fact, psychotics are often outside of discourse, even though they may speak elaborately and wittily. This is because they are not seeking a social bond. However, psychotics may find a way to re-enter discourse through creative or compensatory work, which allows them to remain within it (I will return to this topic in the next chapter). The clinical cases offer us illustrations of symptoms that manifest inside or outside discourse. For example, in cases of conversion hysteria like those of Anna O. or Elizabeth von R., their conversion symptoms were not outside of discourse; they responded to the Hysteric's discourse in opposition to that of the Master. They were addressed to the Other by their interpretability and their objection to the Master's desire. However, that which is referred to by Lacan as psychosomatic phenomena, are outside of discourse since they do not seem to provide a way in which the signifiers and the positions of the elements are clearly accommodated within a discourse, they do not deliver any meaning. Additionally, the fact that psychosomatic phenomena are holophrases[2] suggests that they resist any kind of signification and do not reveal any knowledge (S_2) about a disfigured or cyphered discourse (Lacan, 1964, p. 237).

Discourse is how individuals become subjects, not simply by being subject to language (*langue*), like a parrot or automaton that repeats what it hears. Individuals do not become subjects through echolalia, the mindless repetition of what they hear. Individuals become subjects when they can maneuver speech to signify their own lack, take up a subject-position in relation to their symptoms, and intervene in the significant events of their lives. This happens when they confront and assume their lack, which is a result of their loss of jouissance. The remains of this loss, the lost object (objet petit *a*), separates the individual's needs from their demands, requests, and messages to the Other. When this happens, the subject becomes aware

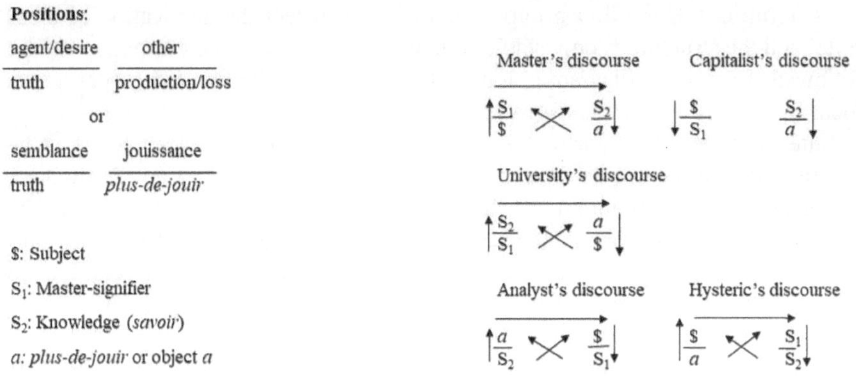

Figure 11.1

of their lack and enters into the metonymy of desire, becoming a subject of desire (Lacan, 1958).

Second, discourse allows us to fill the constitutive void (the Thing) while still using what remains from our encounter with the first Other, mediated by the caregiver. In Chapter 3, we analyzed the first loss, which occurs when we introduce negation into the judgment of existence. Badiou (2005) writes that "there is no language without negation" (p. 335). However, the individual must also experience a second loss, the loss of an imaginary object, which creates a symbolic lack symbolized by Φ, or castration. This allows Lacan to introduce a fourth element in the algebraic formulas of the discourses: the lost object, which operates as the gain of a certain satisfaction, the surplus of enjoyment or object petit *a*. For Lacan, discourse determines the ways in which desire can be tied to the object, that is, in what way it can be desired and to what portion of that surplus-jouissance we will have access in relation to the other and the law. Now, these four elements (S_1, S_2, $, *a*) can be arranged and start to belong to that great set that we can call D, that of the discourse {D}. That {D}, whose members are those four elements, is made up of subsets. Lacan identified four discourses in his Seminar 17: the master, the hysteric, the university, and the analyst. Years later, in a lecture at the University of Milan, he proposed a fifth discourse: the capitalist's. However, he did not give this discourse the same status as the others, because it does not produce a social bond.

These five discourses can be arranged in different ways to create substitutable subsets that represent the power relations in C that make X count as Y. The organization of these subsets shown in Figure 11.1 obeys group theory rather than set theory. In group theory, the four discourses can be arranged in the form of a Klein four-group, a group of four different elements, one of which is an identity element, that obeys certain properties.

The Klein four-group is an algebraic structure, which means that it follows certain rules, such as closure, associativity, identity, and invertibility. The four elements of the discourses can be arranged in a squared disposition according to these rules, forming a Klein four-group. The arrows represent the application of these rules, and the structure is only stable so long as the rules and their arrangement are followed. To read the diagram in Figure 11.1, start at the bottom left corner, in the locus of truth, and follow the arrows.

Entering a discourse, particularly that of the Master (which Lacan posits as the central one and the one that has dominated history), means, for any individual, surrendering a way of enjoying, while becoming deprived and enculturated. The Master, the lord, the priest, the legislator, the entrepreneur, and so many figures of domination are veiled behind the Hegelian Master and his relationship with power. The Master demands that we renounce our first object of satisfaction and love. However, loss is not all in negative, because it also leads to a gain (*plus-de-jouir*), a by-product, or surplus, following Marx's term. The {D} implies the {A} or, by extensionality $\{S_1, S_2\}$, where S_1 would intervene upon the battery of signifiers, which is already a network of propositional knowledge (*savoir*), S_2, a universe of discourse. Now that S_1 intervenes in S_2, in the locus of the Other, the subject, \$, arises in the place of truth. When the master-signifier intervenes on the battery of signifiers, a remainder, object *a*, is left behind. This is what Lacan's algebra of discourses shows, with its different positions for conventional elements. If X counts as Y in C, it is because the Master has made it count through the law. To count means to be ordinal and legal, both a logical and a deontological move.

The law is a complex term in Lacanian thought, ranging from the ambiguous use of jurisprudence to the attributed deontic and apophantic powers of performative utterances. These powers are the foundation of any performative utterance. The law is legitimized by the Master's discourse, such as the Covenant or the Hammurabi code. This Master is not necessarily a supernatural or natural figure but Language and language themselves. In Modernity the figure of the master has been displaced from God to the self, or the one who speaks as "I", who considers itself legitimated to speak within a discourse. Thus, the transcendental "I" is whoever speaks as "I" uttering knowledge that conceals truth, departing from S_1.

> This is the I insofar as it is transcendental, but, equally, insofar as it is illusory. [...] The transcendental I is what anyone who has stated knowledge in a certain way harbors as truth, the S_1, the I of the master. It is, very precisely, out of the I identical to itself that the S_1 of the pure imperative is constituted. It is, very precisely, in the imperatives that the I is displayed for they are always in the second person.
>
> The myth of the ideal I, of the I that masters, of the I whereby at least something is identical to itself, namely the speaker....
>
> (Lacan, 1969–1970, pp. 62–63)

Master of oneself (thus the pun in French, *m'être/maître à moi-même*), or the illusion of autonomy and self-control in Modernity, the Master is the subject itself inside this illusion in the double mirroring with the other.

11.3. NotF as the button tie and master-signifier

Searle's proposition, "X counts as Y in C", fails to account for the enunciator who speaks from a discourse when addressing a truth to the Other. Where is the enunciator speaking from? Who occupies the position of the one who declares the sentence? Does the enunciator embody the figure of the master? Do they intend to replace the master, or to impugn or unmask him? In the Master's discourse, the agent's place is S_1, the first signifier, the multiple-one named by it. In Seminar 18, Lacan suggests that in the Analyst's discourse, the product/loss is the paternal function, or S_1 as NotF (Lacan, 1971, pp. 172–173; Verhaeghe, 2006). This is a new displacement by Lacan of what the NotF is, since it now counts as a master-signifier.

In Part 1, I discussed the first body of signifier, a floating signifier with zero value that establishes the law under the gaze and approval of the Father-God of monotheism and the Covenant laws. It is more the result of signification than the entire signifier/signified chain. This idea does not seem to have changed for Lacan until Seminar 18. In this Seminar, Lacan equates the NotF with the master-signifier, which is related to something I have not mentioned yet but that had been present since Seminar 3, *The Psychoses*: the quilting point (*point de capiton*) or button tie (as B. Fink prefers to call it). The point "at which the signified and the signifier are knotted together, between the still floating mass of meanings that are actually circulating between these two characters and the text" (Lacan, 1955–1956, p. 268). A button tie is a sewing stitch used to hold two pieces of fabric together. For Lacan, the signifier NotF is what ensures that the chain of signifiers is anchored to a set of signifieds in a text, but more specifically to another set of signifiers. The self-referentiality of the NotF is what stops the chain of signifiers from straying and metonymically substituting one signifier for another, which would halt the unfolding of speech. In addition to S_1 and S_2, the signifier must function as a number and follow an order (ordinality). This means that the concatenation of S_1 and S_2 generates meaning based on syntax and propositional chaining. There must also be a third element, an X that closes the count and establishes the interval between S_1 and S_2. This third element is the NotF, the metastructure.

The NotF is an instance and a third signifier. It is the body of the empty signifier, which allows the signifying ordered pair to remain a pair. The NotF is the power-set, or P(A), which makes three without itself counting as a third, excluding itself from the count. "The third element, limit, point, or authority, is the one that establishes the interval, where the subject of the unconscious and the object *a* cause of desire reside, which surrounds the drive" (Eidelsztein, 2019, p. 327). The NotF implies this third element as establishing an ordinality and a point of stop to a cardinality, which makes historization, counting, and the mythical possible.

The master-signifier is everything that points to the ego ideal delegated by the Symbolic father and supports a truth that cannot be further supplemented. It closes off speech, blocks the drift of meaning, and orients it. In other words, the master-signifier organizes the degree of truth in my own statements, in relation to the status function. This does not mean that there are no objective or correspondence truths. Rather, all truth is incomplete; it can only be said halfway, and something of it belongs to the Real. The divagations around truth come to a halt at a certain point. Furthermore, truth is "the sister of jouissance", since any logical system is consistent "only by designating its force of effect of incompleteness, where its limit is marked" (Lacan, 1969–1970, p. 67), and within that limit appears jouissance as a residue, the remainder of Language as pure Real.

11.4. The unchaining of meaning in the absence of NotF: Schreber and Aimée

The S_1 dresses up the NotF as a guarantor of meaning, organizing the degree to which meaning is assumed in discourse. This is the locus where an enunciation is stated, acknowledging a subject-position. In decompensated psychosis, this point is not achieved very clearly. For example, in his *Memoirs of My Nervous Illness*, Schreber describes how at times the voices (or he himself, it is unclear) would ask existential questions outside of any apparent context, followed by incomplete or interrupted responses. These questions seem to express the difficulty of finding reasons for things and the loss of a sense of the meaning of events. Schreber's inability to settle on a discourse prevents him from assuming the locus where his surplus jouissance should be fixed. As a result, unanswerable questions overflow: "Why only?", "Why because?", "Why because I?", "Let it be then", "But why?", and so on. There is no possible orientation that guides the discourse or where to locate *a* and S_2. Similar difficulties with discursive assumptions and sense-making figure in Lacan's doctoral thesis case, Aimée.

She was admitted to Sainte-Anne Hospital by Lacan after attacking Huguette Duflos, a famous film and theater actress of the time. She displayed delusional and incoherent ideas from the moment she arrived at the police station. Her medical history included hospitalizations for persecutory ideas, such as the sensation of being insulted or accused of extraordinary vices in the street. She also had a history of delusions of persecution, jealousy, interpretation, grandeur, erotomania, illusions, and morbid hallucinations. Psychosis first manifested at age 28, during her first pregnancy, and led to hospitalization. She believed that her work colleagues criticized and slandered her, and that newspapers talked about or alluded to her. She imagined people gossiping or making obnoxious comments as they passed her by. She wondered why she was being targeted, but of course found no answer.

After giving birth to a stillborn daughter, she wondered why it had happened. Was someone responsible for her daughter's death? She received an answer from a friend she hadn't spoken to in a long time, who called her shortly after the baby was born dead. She found the call suspicious, but didn't pursue the idea further. Soon after, she became pregnant again and gave birth to a boy, to whom she devoted herself tirelessly. Once again, however, questions, interpretations, and anxiety encroached upon her. Becoming a mother seemed to disturb her anew. It was unclear what these thoughts were, but they must have been questions, impressions, and experiences of jouissance that invaded her in an asemantic fashion (Lacan called them “elementary phenomena”) (Lacan, 1932, 1955–1956). Her fear for her baby’s safety consumed her, believing that her neighbors, motorists, and everyone else was trying to harm him. At the request of her family, she was committed to a hospital, especially after they learned of her plan to flee to the United States to become a famous novelist, even if it meant abandoning her child to save him.

In the interviews with Lacan, the unanswered questions, this lack of assumption of the meaning of what she lived, were condensed into the need behind all to unmask the enemy’s identity, together with a megalomaniac question, “Isn’t she meant to fulfill an exceptional destiny?” (Lacan, 1932).

These questions presupposed a commitment to individuation. They not only outlined a destination that one is forced to seek in the modern world, but also the relationship that this destiny entails with respect to others, one’s peers. What role does the other play in one’s life purpose? What role does the other play in the context of motherhood and having a child?

Aimée’s sexuality and reputation were on everyone’s lips, which made her uneasy because her pregnancy confirmed her sexual activity to others. Additionally, there were the other women: identifications of herself, a feminine ideal projected onto Huguette Duflos, her persecutor, who not only threatened to harm her son but also represented the unfolding of femininity of all the “actresses” with whom she believed her husband slept.

> The lovers that Aimée successively imputes to her husband are, as her delusion progresses, the same ones that her unconscious love designates to her delusional hatred. [...] But Freud demonstrated quite well that properly paranoic delusions of jealousy translate an unconscious sexual attraction towards the accused accomplice, and this applies from start to finish to Aimée’s delusion.
>
> (Lacan, 1932, p. 264 [*Translated by the author*])

The *I* of the paranoic is a fragmented one; as indicated by Freud (1911), it can be decomposed like the Imaginary other can also be. It is an I that projects the reverse image of itself onto others. The psychotic is the paradigm of the subject who lacks mastery over itself, and it is there where the illusion of “being master of oneself” more easily fades, indicating the essential breakdown of agency in the speaking subject. The definition that Lacan seeks to give of the big Other in Seminar 2 is quite indicative of the phenomenon of deep depersonalization and fragmentation of the *I* that the psychotic experiences. Speaking of the objects that the subject encounters, they fall under the weight of an unsurmountable wall, the wall of Language.

> In other words, we in fact address A_1, A_2, those we do not know, true Others, true subjects. [...] Fundamentally, it is them I’m aiming at each time I utter true speech, but I always attain a_1, a_2... I always aim at true subjects, and I have to be content with shadows.
>
> (Lacan, 1954–1955, p. 244)

Shadows, false egos, or the reverse of the ego are the only objects that the psychotic subject is confronted with when the father function falters and seems to fall apart; this is when discourse is not solidly attached by a S_1. The predominance of metonymy as a "sliding of sense" (*glissement du sens*) does not allow the fixation of meaning in a signifier or a series of signifiers. As suggested by E. Pluth (2007), based on a comment by Lacan on a case of Wernicke's aphasia (Lacan, 1955–1956, p. 219), the subject in his statements wanted to release an effect of meaning, but it was not incarnated anywhere; he was trapped in a metonymic stray. In this case, the implementation of the NotF signifier favors the production of a meaning effect. "Even though metaphor, in contrast to metonymy, achieves 'verbal incarnation' of meaning, a meaning is still not fully, or simply, present in it" (Pluth, 2007, p. 38). Metaphor needs the metonymy of the signifying chain. However, the meaning (signified effect) produced in any speech is something that is not necessarily contained within the signifying chain; instead it resonates within it, passing to the big Other through the intermediate of the small other without ever really reaching a full effect. The decompensated psychotic cannot make resonate within the small other a message sustaining the social bond that returns from the Other.

The lack of that S_1 to trace Aimée's path contrives the intimate confusion and existential drift in which she finds herself. The $\{S_2\}$ will be left without a point of reference to guide the discursive circuit due to the lack of that button tie (*point de capiton*), generating the slippage of meaning without anything anchoring it. This is characteristic of the triggering phases of psychosis when the subject is confronted with a "void of meaning" and perplexity, the instantiation moment of foreclosure of the NotF. These are seen in Schreber before his second psychotic outbreak in 1893: sleeplessness, anxiety, hypochondriac ideas, hyperesthesias, and cenesthopathies. The rupture of the button tie leads to a disarticulation of meaning and bodily experience in the psychotic. The body is experienced as something that is no longer linked to words or meaning (Londoño, 2017). Faced with the Thing opening its jaws and generating the anxiety-laden perplexity that the psychotic experiences with the disordered movement of the signifier, she must look for a possible closure, something that once again cloaks the presentation of the Thing. The construction of delusion, or the delusional metaphor, is what most frequently comes at hand for the psychotic.

The modern subject bases its actions and sayings on the discourse of the master, the university, the hysteric, or the capitalist because these discourses can be historicized and account for the events of everyday life that the Imaginary other leaves unspoken and unresolved. The ontology of social facts implies the assent or dissent of the other to one's actions and utterances, but this Imaginary other often leaves us hanging. Our statements remain unanswered or misrepresented, and some of the addressed message is lost. However, the neurotic who talks can assume that there is a kernel of truth in the Imaginary other that can be returned to it, and that a desire interrogates it from the other side where object *a* is found. Even if psychotics take refuge in discourses such as the University's (as Gödel and Cantor did) or the Master's (as Hitler did), they cannot guarantee their place as I (*je*), as a statement shifter (in the linguistic sense). Their utterances will always fall into a void of bewilderment.

Following the question that I indicated at the end of Chapter 4 and that Lacan formulated as the ultimate question, "what am I?" (Lacan, 1960, p. 694), the psychotic remains muddled up with it, especially regarding the problem of jouissance and the scope of its own statements regarding a desire that does not appear on the horizon beyond itself, in the locus of the Other.

Notes

1 The master-signifier and the term signifier in Lacan should not be limited in definition to a single word, or to a correspondence with a word or a term. A signifier could mean a proposition or a propositional attitude, thus, a belief, a desire, or an intention that can be uttered in an articulated manner. Now, a master-signifier is the minimum propositional set or metastructure that allows quilting or tying up the whole sequence of referral allowing to stop the incessant production of meaning by closing the loop at a spot.

2 Lacan considers holophrases as "phrases, expressions which cannot be broken down, and which have to be related to a situation taken in its entirety..." (Lacan, 1953–1954, p. 225). In linguistics it's a signifier employed in a way that expresses more than itself, referring to a more complex situation, or that means way more than it evokes on its own.

12

The outside-discourse of psychosis

A bet on subjectivization and the fundamental fantasy

12.1. The discourse and the constitution of the social bond

Power operates through discourse to regulate the sexes, jouissance, and the law. For Lacan, discourse is a form that "inscribes our conduct, possibly our acts, within the framework of certain primordial statements" (Lacan, 1969–1970, p. 13). It is a structural framework of intersubjective relations that favors the regulation of jouissance and desire between speaking beings. Discourse is not simply speech, but the established typical forms of relations between individuals organized by the language structure. Thus, discourse sustains the social bond (*lien social*). Lacan suggests that the question of the social bond, of what allows an individual subject to engage with a community of reference, is precisely formulated when the individual disengages from the norms of collectivity. How does the subject manage its bond and relationship with the other? As Marie-Jean Sauret asks, the question is not how we stick together with those with whom we have a reciprocal, kind relationship, but with those we consider alien, different, or dangerous (Sauret, 2009).

The transition to Modernity's individualism established a new discourse that threw individuals into a void of meaning regarding their own existence. This new discourse forced them to assume an unprecedented responsibility for their own destiny, with only the fragile support of their faith in God and the mundane chores of everyday life. Anglo-Saxon Puritanism and Calvinism, in particular, de-idealized a life consecrated to religious rituals, promulgating instead the virtue of worldly existence and the attachment to labor.

On the one hand, Cartesianism and Protestantism's postulates confronted us with the horror of emptiness and uncertainty. On the other hand, a superegoic force seems to attract us towards a face-to-face encounter with unbearable jouissance and the Thing. On the edge of the void, how does the modern individual defend itself against these distressing truths and the inescapable reality of its loneliness, which seems to lead to its own ruin? Modernity leaves individuals immensely vulnerable, with no Other to provide support or meaning. This individual must construct a big Other beyond what its immediate caregivers and community can offer, or what it itself seems to embody. However, this Other will be as inconsistent and

DOI: 10.4324/9781032663616-16

uncertain as the one that Modernity buried, even though it is the only semblance of an Other that the individual can rely on.

12.2. What is being outside of discourse?

In his 1972 work *L'étourdit*, Lacan argues that psychoanalysis must deal with the truth beyond the proposition, specifically with the absence of the sexual relation. However, an interpretation aiming at truth can still be reached through the proposition, even though the psychoanalyst must sometimes deal with the "outside-discourse of psychosis" (Lacan, 1972, p. 490). Lacan does not elaborate on this revealing phrase, but it allows us to continue with our approach. In the same text, Lacan suggests that the schizophrenic does not receive any aid from discourse, leaving them disarmed and facing the problem of having a body (Lacan, 1972, p. 474). Thus, the psychotic appears to be outside discourse, a strong statement but very guiding for understanding the signifier NotF. It means being outside the ways in which discourse represents both a background and a network of meanings and functional positions assumed, especially where the Other is included as a possible interlocutor and legitimizer of the truth of one's own utterances. While not totally outside, psychoses are delimited by what NotF favors in its Symbolic and formative inscription of the subject. Even if foreclosure of the signifier does not prevent the subject from using language correctly, even obsessively and elaborately, it does favor a fall into an enigma, a void regarding the reason for their own existence, to which the psychotic seems to succumb wretchedly. This can be seen in philosophers such as Charles S. Peirce and J.J. Rousseau, writers such as James Joyce and Philip K. Dick, and theater and poetry artists such as Antonin Artaud and Friedrich Hölderlin. However, some of these authors managed to conceive a supplementary device[1] (*suppléance*) around their uses of the signifier and their containment of jouissance through writing and intellectual lucubration, allowing for long-lasting stabilizations.

Can being outside of discourse constitute a social bond? Psychotics in crisis, who are fully decompensated and usually require hospitalization, are totally cut off from the social bond and thus are outside of discourse. One can infer that stabilized or compensated psychotics are also incapable of genuine and lasting social relationships, or have only unstable relationships or a strong dependence on others. Alternatively, they may only be able to occupy the place of a Master.

However, the compensated and the stabilized psychotic subjects can remain within the social bond and partially inside discourse. Their ways of enjoying may not fully fit in with the social bond, or they may divorce from it completely. To identify how someone finds their way of enjoying and desiring, one can rely on their fundamental fantasy. The latter is a concept that refers to a point reached in an analysis. It can sometimes be identified in certain subjects through their testimonies and the presence of an "indelible image" (Maleval, 2019). This is a fantasized or recalled scene that remains fixed, is experienced as a concrete reality, and compresses jouissance. In psychosis, these images frame jouissance in a rigid, non-phallic way, precariously veil the drive object (object *a*), and seem to fix one's own jouissance in a particular way that largely defines many of the actions in the subject's life (Maleval, 2019). It is the best possible way for the Imaginary to cover the Real, but its Symbolic consistency is very precarious due to the lack of the NotF.

12.3. The indelible images and the place of the fundamental fantasy in psychosis

Psychoanalyst J.-C. Maleval suggests that the psychotic does not count with a fundamental fantasy, or that the closest thing to it is an indelible image, a semblance of the fundamental fantasy. This means that unlike the psychotic, the neurotic subject's position is determined by its desire, its response to demand, and the meaning of its need. This meaning is not related to the scenario in which any such fantasy may interfere, but comes from the Other. In other words, the neurotic subject attributes the meaning of the demand to the Other. Fundamental fantasy traces the limits of being and confronts the subject to wonder about the lack in which it appears to itself as desire, by carrying demand to the limits of being (Lacan, 1958a, p. 533). The actions of speaking beings, supported by their desire and the chains of signifiers, take place against the backdrop and frame of reference of the fundamental fantasy. For example, even though the status of willful actions in neurosis is hazy, they are not exempt from the fundamental fantasy. Lacan's graph of desire shows that the neurotic symptom is a metaphor that is supposed to start at S(Ⱥ) and pass through the fantasy ($ ◊ *a*) to reach the signified of the Other, s(A). This inscribes the symptomatic metaphor as the substitution of one signifier for another (Lacan, 1960). The fundamental fantasy formula ($ ◊ *a*), briefly mentioned in Chapter 3, means that the divided subject is in a relationship with object *a*, that is, they are both involved and developed, or both conjoined and disjoined. The left side of the diamond (◊) represents what relies on the subject, while the right side represents what occurs in or is attributed to the Other. The fundamental fantasy simply indicates how a subject relates to the Other and to the desire and the jouissance that are placed in the Other (object *a*, the cause of desire)[2]. This fantasy can be identified as a word in a statement, or a simple declaration made by an analysand during analysis, as a background script, or as an image described in a diary, narrative, etc. In any case, it can be something as simple as a stated proposition.

> The plethora of intrusive thoughts, scenarios, daydreams [and dreams], and masturbation fantasies any one subject has are thus viewed by Lacan as essentially permutations of the fundamental fantasy, usually presenting one facet of that fundamental fantasy. To put it differently, the countless intrusive thoughts, scenarios, daydreams, and masturbation fantasies are theorized to boil down or cook down to a 'single' fundamental fantasy.
>
> (Fink, 2014, p. 44)

Hysterical and obsessive-neurotic subjects have a specific way of accommodating themselves in relation to the Other and their own lack, object *a* (see Fink, 1997, Ch. 8). Ultimately, the fundamental fantasy outlines how any subject interprets the desire of the Other, its place in the world, and its apprehension of reality. As Sauret (2009) indicates, a discourse is only inhabitable if it complements or replaces fantasy. The discourse in which a subject is positioned, articulated to this fundamental fantasy, is necessary to maintain some form of social bond, and full jouissance and the encounter with the Thing at a distance.

In the formation of the fundamental fantasy in psychosis, something seems to malfunction, leaving its articulation incomplete. Maleval suggests that the indelible image of someone like Schreber could be portrayed in the sudden thought that triggered his delusional drift: "...it really must be rather pleasant to be a woman succumbing to intercourse" (Schreber, 2000, p. 46). Is this just a delusional idea or the simplest statement closest to a fundamental fantasy? Distinguishing between the indelible image and the fundamental fantasy is not easy, and the two seem to overlap. In psychosis, the indelible image and its statement operate as something persecutory; their underlying intentions come from the Other of jouissance, not from the subject itself. This places the subject in the position of a passive object, subject to an imposition of "an invasive jouissance, not negativized, [from which] a lack of operationalization of the limiting function of the phallus is deduced", and the emergence of the indelible images "testifies to a failure of repression and a predominance of the Imaginary, even a certain inability to provide the subject with a consistent 'substance' [étoffe]" (Maleval, 2019, p. 143). The fundamental fantasy in psychosis seems to falter, failing to provide a true consistency to the locus of the Other and the mystery of its desire. For the psychotic, this weakness of the fundamental fantasy deprives it of "an engine of psychic reality, that of the divided subject", or as Maleval expresses it, a compass that guides the subject in its existence. The fundamental fantasy's assumption depends on the inscription of the NotF, the extraction of object *a*, and its projection onto the locus of the Other. A subject with a psychotic structure may experience itself as empty, emotionless, and fraudulent, as if the facts of life lacked authenticity. This makes it more susceptible to encountering the Thing and the Other jouissance[3]. Additionally, it does not experience jouissance in a way that allows it to adjust the pleasure principle or feel that it is participating in the process of seeking the object as an S_1 linked to an S_2.

Maleval uses various examples, both clinical and literary, to refer to these indelible images. One example is the writer and essayist Yukio Mishima, who in his autobiographical work, *Confessions of a Mask*, discloses a necrophiliac and sadistic orientation of his jouissance. After seeing the painting *The Martyrdom of Saint Sebastian* by Guido Reni at a young age, Mishima experienced a vivid excitement that led to other fantasies involving murdered young princes with whom he fell in love, as well as a fascination with images of torture and human sacrifice that haunted him from an early age. In his literary work, Maleval alludes to his tragic end—an apotheotic death that materializes when he asks his lover to decapitate him after performing hara-kiri following the failed coup he organized with a militia. He figures the Other of jouissance as the recipient of his sacrificial gift. His death should restore world order, order in Japan, the emperor, and the country's glory.

> The martyrdom of Saint Sebastian… seems to have allowed Mishima to aestheticize his sacrificial position. It is after being organized by what the specialists called "a necrophiliac aesthetic" that his important written work, articulated to the indelible image, could serve for a long time as a supplementary device [*suppléance*].
>
> (Maleval, 2019, p. 152)

Another case is that of Nelson Cooper, reported in the book *The Breathless Orgasm*, about the masturbatory practice of self-asphyxiation (Money, Wainwright, and Hinsburger, 1991). Cooper required fantasizing about young women and men being strangled to reach orgasm. From a young age, he began the practice of self-choking based on an indelible image of a "woman trying to escape death" or "a woman being strangled". It was while watching movies and television that these images came to him as a framework for his own jouissance. The masturbatory practice often contained an aspect of transitivism since he pictured himself as the victim of a homosexual man who strangled him, and he did this while choking himself with a pair of pantyhose to the point of almost losing consciousness, immediately letting himself fall to the ground like if it were the body dropping dead. After that, he masturbated until reaching orgasm; this practice was performed many times a day, about 12 to 14 times. He thought he was losing his mind, feeling compelled to take a life-threatening risk, but only this could somewhat contain his overflowing jouissance. This routine stopped him from having loving relationships with women, which he strongly wanted. It became so disturbing that he went to the police station one day to ask to be hospitalized. He appeared in these masturbatory fantasies as the object of the jouissance of an evil *jouisseur* (enjoyer), to whom he exposed as waste.

12.4. The psychotic structure beyond the clinical signs

The topic of the indelible images extends to Lacan's concept of the "psychotic structure", suggesting that psychosis can be identified beyond the explicit phenomena of a psychotic crisis, such as decompensation and onsets that require hospitalization. This raises the question: Can psychosis be thought of outside of these explicit phenomena? Lacan's proposal of untriggered psychosis or pre-psychosis imply a type of psychosis that either never develops into a full-blown psychotic crisis or that develops without any obvious trigger or clear-cut manifestation. This hypothesis is a reminder to clinicians not to limit their practice to observable clinical signs, and to take necessary precautions in psychoanalysis to avoid triggering a psychotic breakout. "There is nothing that more closely resembles a neurotic symptomatology than prepsychotic symptomatology" (Lacan, 1955–1956, p. 191).

Neurotics, like psychotics, can also construct an external reality or pseudoreality. Fantasy is important in neurosis, and for Lacan, it is not far removed from delusion in psychosis. Based on the clinical cases of Maurits Katan (1950) and Helene Deutsch (2007), Lacan identified a type of neurotic subject with an absent Oedipus complex and a foreclosed NotF. Deutsch called these subjects "as-if personalities" because they could easily pass for ordinary neurotics but were prone to imaginary compensations, superficial identifications, and deep emotional disturbances. This means, subjects that do not really enter the game of the signifier, or "a non-integration… into the register of the signifier" (Lacan, 1955–1956, p. 251). Lacanian psychoanalysts have been grappling with the question of how to diagnose psychosis outside of its obvious signs, such as delusions, hallucinations, negative symptoms, and disorganized thought. The debate has been rich and varied, but I will not go into detail here (for a deeper understanding, I recommend reading Redmond, 2014 or Vanheule, 2019). However, Lacan himself provides a clue in his Seminar *The Psychoses*. He suggests that the psychotic's experience of exteriority or dispossession in relation to the Other (A) may indicate that they have never fully entered into Language (Lacan, 1955–1956, p. 250). In Language, the psychotic subject has undoubtedly entered, but perhaps it would be more accurate to say that they have not fully assumed a subject-position with respect to discourse and the treatment of loss or surplus of jouissance; or that they come to live as inhabited by Language, as objects of Language themselves (see section 8.4). This may be due to a rigid assumption of the subject-position that is not guided by the phallic and paternal signifiers, or to a treatment of loss or surplus that is carried out on their own body or without regard for the Other, leading to egocentrism, megalomania, utilitarianism, etc. Or it could be that the lack of lack pushes them to a problem of assuming their own body and that of the Other. In any case, the psychotic subject has difficulty assuming a subject-position that is guided by the NotF, the Symbolic function of the father.

12.5. The specificity of desire in psychosis

To understand the psychotic subject's relationship to surplus-jouissance, knowledge (S_2), and the master-signifier (S_1), it is important to consider the semblance of discourse on which they stand. This is the S_1 that can superficially occupy the foreclosed NotF if a work of "recovery" or "reconstruction" is operating, as indicated by Freud's discussion of the delusions of the paranoic. Once this is understood, questions about object *a* and S_1 become more pressing. Lacanian analysts have long neglected the topic of desire in psychosis, assuming either that it is absent due to the lack of NotF or that it is not of interest in clinical cases. Most texts focus on how to set boundaries for deregulated jouissance, ignoring the peculiar way in which the psychotic deals with desire (De Battista, 2017). According to J. de Battista, in psychosis, desire does not appear symbolized by the NotF; it would not be traversed by the phallus as a signifier of the lack, "[t]hat is, a desire that is not knotted to the law of the father, dimension that characterizes the position of the psychotic as one of rejection of the paternal imposture. The desire of the psychotic would not be sealed by the consent of the father" (De Battista, 2017, p. 2). Desire is a condition, as Lacan and De Battista remind us, not a consequence of the introduction of the Law.

> For far from giving myself over to some logicizing reduction where desire is at stake, I detect in desire's irreducibility to demand the very mainspring of what also prevents it from being reduced to need. To put it elliptically: it is precisely because desire is articulated that it is not articulable—by which I mean in the discourse that suits it, an ethical, not a psychological discourse.
>
> [...]
>
> But I will stop here again in order to return to the status of desire, which presents itself as independent of the Law's mediation, because Law originates in desire—owing to the fact that, by an odd symmetry, desire reverses the unconditionality of the demand for love, in which the subject remains subjected to the Other, in order to raise it to the power of an absolute condition (in which "absolute" also implies "detachment").
>
> (Lacan, 1960, pp. 681, 689)

Psychoanalysis views desire and prohibition as inextricably linked. Once the ego enters the world of law, it becomes subservient to the superego and the id. This means that prohibition does not necessarily preclude satisfaction. For example, a toddler may be denied a way to find satisfaction, creating a lack. However, the possibility of seeking a legitimized satisfaction is now structurally and logically open. Desire, in psychoanalysis, is precisely this: a prohibition implies an opening towards a concession, which is where desire lies. Lacan links desire to the Tenth Commandment in the *Ethics* Seminar, establishing a clear connection between it and the Law (Lacan, 1959–1960, pp. 82–83; see section 7.2).

In principle, Lacan originally argued that desire is the cause of the Law, rather than the other way around. Desire cannot be reduced to a demand for love, which all demands are, and it favors detachment from the Other. The Law of the Father is therefore the absolute condition under which desire can or cannot fall. Lacan indicated that the introduction of this law is necessary to bridle the appearance of the Other's omnipotence. For the toddler, detachment from the Other favors the extraction of object *a*, which can take the form of Winnicott's "transitional object". This also leads to the implementation of the structure of fantasy (Lacan, 1960, p. 689). However, in the Seminar *Anxiety*, Lacan equates desire and the law as barriers to accessing the Thing (Lacan, 1962–1963, p. 81).

What are the implications for the "outside-discourse" of psychosis if desire is not knotted to the Law of the Father or sealed by the Father's consent? Could it be a desire that is never supported by discourse and that does not find a place in any of the four positions (agent, truth, etc.) offered by the mathemes[4] of discourse? I will try to describe what happens in the case of the fundamental fantasy, the guide and script of the courses of desire.

The mathemes of the discourses show how the formula of the fundamental fantasy can be accommodated within some discourses but not others. In particular, fantasy does not seem to fit in the Master's discourse. In the Capitalist's discourse, on the other hand, fantasy starts from object *a* in the place of surplus-jouissance or from the product going towards the semblance, \$. In the classic Master's discourse, the master orders a containment of pleasures and jouissance and grants the slave certain rights and duties. This implies that the slave must renounce absolute jouissance in exchange for a more-or-less assured life, resigning itself to whatever the master decides.

On the other hand, and cross-referring to Figure 11.1, fantasy does not seem to be taken into account in this discourse; in any case, the object *a*, instead of product or *plus-de-jouir*, is addressed to the semblance or agent, which in this case is the master-signifier, S_1, whereas the subject addresses knowledge (S_2) directly as an other, without any intermediary. No truth reaches the subject; the agent is already the supposed and unquestionable truth in itself. The arrow that goes upwards supposes that the subject (\$) starts as truth towards S_1 and towards S_2; they are not the ones that condition or delimit, but it is the agent who establishes them. Lacan explains that the essence of the Master's discourse is that the master does not know what he really wants, but that it is the slave who really knows what the master wants. Meanwhile, the master dominates knowledge, S_2, the all-knowing, or the tyranny of knowledge (Lacan, 1969–1970, p. 32).

In the Master's discourse, the Other and jouissance are reduced to knowledge that is used to produce objects, metonymic displacements of object *a*. The slave must produce what the master orders, who stands on a pedestal of all-knowingness but does not consider the slave's or their own fundamental fantasy, ignoring their own subjective division. It is important to remember that the agent in the Master's discourse is nothing more than a semblance of the master, always lacking and insufficient, no matter how hard they try to hide it. Revealing one's fundamental fantasy and the desire of the Other is what makes the Master's project fail when they put themselves in the place of an absolute, especially in psychotic subjects. We can see this in many leaders of religious cults, whose projects end in failure when their followers discover that the emperor had no clothes. Unfortunately, things sometimes end in tragedy.

12.6. The two poles (and a middle ground) of desire and the Master's discourse in psychosis: three vignettes

In the absence of a lack that drives desire, the Other may offer the psychotic a shaky support of identification. However, the psychotic will easily succumb to this irrevocable image when these identifications break. On the one hand, there are two poles of untriggered psychosis or seemingly compensated psychosis that can arise from the predominant discourse, that of the Master, and the position one assumes within it. The first pole consists of those subjects who embody the absolute master and the full scope of the agent, a rigid master-signifier. Their megalomaniac, eccentric, and egocentric visions are experienced as an imperative that they must fulfill, and their desire is not guided by a fantasy that serves as a frame and legal limit of the Other's body and jouissance. The transgressions and submission of the Other to the absolute will of the master and his knowledge completely crush the Other who follows him, placing this Other as the pure object of his drive satisfaction This is evident in the case of Jim Jones, leader of the cult *People's Temple.* Jones shrewdly manipulated his followers into doing whatever he asked, ranging from sexual favors of all kinds, to handing over all their possessions and money, to sacrificing their own lives. He demanded complete fulfillment and release of jouissance from the Other, considering himself a god or deity on Earth. Fantasies of death and domination over the lives of others were a constant in Jones' life from an early age. His father was a veteran of the Great War, disabled by a gas attack, diminished, and unable to work, depending on a meager military pension. He turned into a man who spent his days drinking in a bar while his wife provided for the family. Little Jim Jones grew up on the streets of his hometown without any supervision. His father was absent, and his mother, while providing for him, had no issue with letting him wander the streets all day while she was at the factory. Several witnesses recalled never witnessing any signs of affection or tenderness exchanged between Jones and his parents. He seemed to grow up in an environment where the place of the Father and the Law conveyed by the maternal speech appeared totally decimated.

From a young age, Jim Jones saw preaching and ministry as a way to deal with the Other, in a complete disregard of any sincere desire for the Other within a true social bond. He was known for mistreating and killing animals, often performing funeral rites for them with other children in attendance; he managed to convince them to attend to these funeral performances. At 17, he worked as a hospital orderly, moving corpses and waste without any sign of displeasure. It was while preparing the corpse of a pregnant woman that he met his wife, a nursing student. From that age he felt a great attraction for preaching and communism, imagining an ideal world of social and racial equality, a multiracial congregation of real cooperative interactions. He had been introduced into the world of religion and proselytism of the word of God through a lady neighbor who took care of him when he used to roam in the streets. Thanks to her, he started attending religious ceremonies, masses of several Christian inclinations, and began learning the manners, the proper speeches, the biblical catch-phrases, and the charming behaviors of the preachers while captivating their public. It was his introduction into the world of ministry and the place of the master where he saw the possibility of tracing an ego-ideal.

Jones possessed remarkable oratory skills, often able to persuade others, yet he grew furious and daunting when met with resistance or disobedience. His aspiration seemed centered on forging a cult of personality and the position of absolute Master, marked by megalomaniac notions that influenced how he interacted with his followers within the cult he had established. Many years later, once he had his large congregation of parishioners, on several occasions he deceived them into believing that they had been fed poison and were going to die. He wanted to know how far they were willing to go for him. He didn't care about misleading them, making them think that he had divine powers of healing, mind reading, and even resurrection of the dead. Astonishingly, he orchestrated two assassination attempts with his closest acolytes, feigning his miraculous recovery each time. Furthermore, it remains uncertain whether Jones was performing or genuinely convinced, yet he insisted the congregation faced danger. External entities, particularly the FBI and CIA, were after them according to him, issuing threats to dismantle and obliterate the group. They supposedly had tapped the congregation's phones and placed microphones at the meeting centers (Guinn, 2017).

The master-signifier "congregation", with which a religious community is commonly defined, was for Jones his ideal point; intending to turn his efforts into a "multiracial congregation". He also demanded being called "Father" by his parishioners, but this signifier was devoid of meaning. Both master-signifiers had a neological value for him, where his peers were not subjects with their own particular lack and subjectivity, which counted as the ends of his intentions, but only as the means within a project of infatuation and absolute senseless loyalty. In this construct, individual differences dissolved, merging into a sole devotion to Jones and his cause. However, these master-signifiers were still an ideal but that was not based on the law of NotF and the symbolic covenant, as their signified did not remit to other signifiers in the field of the Other. If he demanded being called Father, this signifier was nothing more than a hollow semblance, a ruse for the Other, with a private, solipsistic, and unattainable meaning. To be the Father meant for Jones that anything was allowed for him, including deception, abuse, physical punishment to disobedience, and threats to deserters, to the point of forcing suicide in order to keep the congregation united under his command. If that is what a Father was meant to do in order to maintain unity and obedience, then it had to be done. On the other hand, the shared meaning of "congregation" or "community" counted only as a means where one's duty to help one's peers, historically disadvantaged ethnic groups, was mixed with an imperative to keep everyone under tension at any cost, under the mantle of that same imperative of "having to remain united". Hence, any threat to unity was repressed and severely punished. In a way, for Jones the only truth for being and sustaining the ideal resided in a coerced choice: total unity *or* death, no middle grounds.

Thus, the Other was not an end but a means for the fulfillment of this urge towards death that had always accompanied him, a possible indelible image of an insistent jouissance. Obviously, as is well known, this is how the fate of *People's Temple* ends up being welded: in the largest collective suicide in history. Now, why settle his behaviors, attitudes, and relations with the Other in a discourse of absolute mastery? Leaders with a psychotic structure, such as Jones, cult personalities, certain politicians, entrepreneurs, and mob bosses, do not project their desire onto the Other. Instead, they see the Other as an object to be used, a source of usufruct. This can lead to attachment, identification, or the use of the Other as a compensating point. This gives us a clue about how to think about love and relationships in psychosis. Unlike the pervert, the psychotic lives the jouissance of the Other as a persecutory imperative or a drive demand, as something that seems to surpass it, while the former seeks the division or anxiety of the Other in jouissance. For Jones, anyone who served as an object for his cause was acceptable, as long as they paid devotion and tribute. The urge towards death was the triumphant closure of a revolutionary act, a mass suicide, where the objects of jouissance slid and multiplied outside of any social bond, completely desubjectivizing the Other.

At the other pole of untriggered psychoses inside the Master's discourse, we have subjects who are annulled, totally introverted, and desperately in need of a "master"—but not to impugn him, like the hysteric. This places them in the Master's discourse, not even in the place of the slave, but in the place of the proletarian, completely helpless and lacking knowledge. These subjects are confused, disoriented, and lack desire. They resort to all kinds of precarious identifications in order to give consistency to their being and their body. Perhaps the most representative case is that of the young woman, the daughter of a family of European nobility, presented by H. Deutsch (2007). This psychoanalyst explains how this young woman grew up without any gesture of tenderness or love from her parents, being raised by nurses but never really feeling any affection, desire, or love, neither for them nor for her parents. The fantasies that she occasionally had where she saw herself with a family were not for the purpose of obtaining any longing for love or token of affection but for obtaining narcissistic benefits. Those fantasized parents were very distant from the real ones and did not match a possible Oedipus complex with them. When she was older, those fantasies disappeared and other equally narcissistic fantasies arose, but she had to identify with another person to be able to act on them. When she was at school, she acted like the other classmates to conform to the norm; friendships meant nothing to her; she prayed and acted as if she were a believer, but she did not feel the slightest religious fervor; and she behaved in a standard way but only by imitating the others. The NotF signifier was inoperative in her; the Law of the Father never really seemed to have applied to her, which meant that an intrapsychic conflict between the drives and the objects of the world did not arise. If there was no immediate parent figure to tell her that something was not to be done, she would proceed without much inconvenience. Hence, later in her life, she lent herself without question or by inertia to participate in alcohol intakes, cults, artistic and political movements, perverse sexual activities, etc. She did all of this without feeling guilt or the slightest conviction in what she was performing; she simply followed the whims of the Other, who indicated where she should go and do. Her desire depended on the master's, slipping and multiplying without any apparent button tie, like an object hauled along by the slippage of the master-signifier of the Other. It is peculiar that the Other was not a persecutory agent, but that she instead submitted and surrendered herself to its jouissance.

What common features do these two poles of the psychotic structure share? How can we identify the foreclosure of the NotF? In both cases, we can identify the absence of the button tie or quilting point that ties desire to the Law. On the other hand, the absence of fundamental fantasy and the non-extraction of object *a* are also evident. In both poles, taking refuge in discourse, particularly the Master's, is a way to solve structural impasses, such as the lack of the paternal metaphor, and to maneuver jouissance and unbridled drive demands. The Master's discourse replaces the lack of fundamental fantasy, but the psychotic is unable to distance itself from the Master's jouissance.

Finally, in Hervé Castanet's book *Quand le corps se défait*, I find a case that lies between these former poles, a sort of middle ground to the psychotic's response to the Master's discourse. This particular case reveals a concealed psychotic structure beneath what appears to be a straightforward diagnosis. Despite the gravity of the issues the analysand has raised, he has led a life unnoticed by others, not posing problems for those around him. He is witty at concealing his suffering and all that it encompasses from those closest to him.

Séverin, a 40-year-old widower with a six-year-old son, works as a night watchman at an emergency-handling power plant. Since his teenage years, he has excessively indulged in alcohol. His consumption spikes when he feels distressed or anxious, seeking to avoid thinking, escape anxiety, and detach from himself. This often leads to complete unconsciousness or near alcohol-induced comas. Occasionally, he vanishes for entire weekends, leaving his son under the care of family friends or his mother. During these aimless escapades, he drives around, frequents bars, and drinks until memories fade. Upon returning home, once sobered, he remarks on life's stagnancy, feeling trapped in an unchanging present frozen in time.

At work, he admits to doing nothing during long nights—merely sitting on a couch for hours, not reading, watching TV, or even daydreaming. He seems disconnected from both the Other and the world around him. Castanet characterizes this subject's body as

> a body mass [that] remains strange, autonomous, loosened, in short, [R]eal. In the absence of the signifier that would trigger the flesh and allow its appropriation. By proceeding in this way, he even partially obtains a consistency of being. The bodily shocks obtained thanks to alcohol… give him sensations of which he otherwise knows nothing. He holds on to life by mistreating this body which is only his when it receives blows and bears the scars of pain for days on end.
>
> (Castanet, 2017, p. 98 [*Translated by the author*])

The self-destructive behavior has been prevalent for years, even before he met his wife, whose suicide did not seem to surprise him, nor did he seem to question it too much. It is just something he suspected she was going to end up doing; she always preferred death over him and their son. During his psychoanalysis, he does not seek to find meaning in that troubling death; it seems that this suicide for him would have been something meaningless in front of which he runs into a wall. There is, then, nothing to say in front of that insurmountable wall. Death seems to be the constant weight of Séverin's life, the inevitable pit into which he will end up falling. His entire life revolves around mistreating his body, consuming it in a deleterious jouissance of self-destructive repetition, and this deadly compulsion is closely related to what we could classify as an indelible image. Castanet describes a scene when as a child, his mother used to wash his private parts when she suddenly transformed into an opaque and dangerous mass that could strike him and tear him to pieces. According to the psychoanalyst, this indelible image slides metonymically towards any woman, from the mother to any potential partner in his life.

His father, an alcoholic like him whom he had to go look for in bars as a child, figured in Severin's imagination in his violent words of reproach and insults. That man would have been just like him, castrated and devirilized by his mother. For Séverin, his mother would have totally destroyed and consumed his father. He stated that: "*If my father drank, it was because he was not sexually satisfied with my mother. She persecuted him sexually*". The paternal signifier would not have operated as a third mediating instance in the mother-son dyad. "The violence he exercises on himself by destroying his life is that projected onto the father; he is literally him" (Castanet, 2017, p. 109). As I indicated in Chapter 5, the child must go from that Imaginary, absorbing, and fusing relationship with the mother to the encounter with the paternal mediating instance of castration. The paternal phallus and the NotF introduce the child to the lack and open the possibility for something to come into play that allows it to get out of an Imaginary rivalry of "either you or me". All these events would be captured in some invented myth in which the child is introduced to the neurotic structure in some sort of resolution to the maternal desire inside a phobic reaction.

For Castanet, Séverin is a psychotic subject, even though he has never been hospitalized for any crisis, has never been diagnosed by a psychiatrist, or has had to take medication of any kind. Only his general practitioner says that he suffered from depression, and his work colleagues say that he was kind of bizarre. Apart from this and his notable alcoholism, however, Séverin could pass for medical-psychological services simply as that, as an alcoholic who does not manage to cope with his addiction. He would be treated as someone with poor self-control, unable to deal with his personal autonomy, and failing to be master of his own life and actions. However, the problem does not lie in poor self-control or lack of ownership of his life; Séverin knows what he is doing and does not seem to want to stop. Even if he goes to the psychoanalyst to try to remedy something in his life situation, drinking offers him a self-therapeutic possibility and a certain relief. It is perhaps the double-edged sword that has allowed him to sustain in his existence. Prey to that indelible image that hides a destructive and unregulated jouissance, he has lived his life as a victim of a persecuting maternal Other, even though he himself continues to live with his mother, and it is she who pays for his analysis. In addition to feeling as though the feminine-maternal figure is crushing him, he believes that his life has been meaningless and empty, "a disturbance that occurred at the inmost juncture of the subject's sense of life" (Lacan, 1959, p. 466).

After three assiduous years of analysis, Séverin breaks with his analytical cure in an untimely manner, in what Castanet describes as a *passage à l'acte*. He meets a woman with whom he has a relationship. In a phone call he confirms that he is not going to continue with analysis anymore because he has met this woman. However, the call is alarming for Castanet, since Séverin's words do not suggest that this encounter will be experienced as something fortunate but rather as a condemnation and a sentence that will lead to his downfall. That "love at first sight" encounter (in French, *coup de foudre,* literally "lightning strike") that Séverin describes to Castanet is an equivalent of his own destruction. It is, in a literal sense, a strike or a blow to him. During his last session, he asked, "*How far can a man go to be handed over to a woman?*" That is what, according to Castanet, Séverin did: he handed himself to the jouissance of the Other, refusing to be master of himself. In a paradoxical move, he freed himself by delivering his soul to the jouissance of the Other in the guise of "crazy love" (*amour à la folie*).

If no object cause of desire is located or projected onto the Other, the subject itself becomes the object of the Other's jouissance, and its being is reduced to incarnating that object. However, because this discourse does not guarantee the sustainability of the social bond for the psychotic, we can conclude that the psychotic is more outside of discourse than inside of it. In other words, discourse does not offer any assurance to the cohesion of the social bond in psychosis.

Now, the idea of the Real father emerges in the latter vignette as an impossibility, a paradoxical entity that only gains validity through its symbolic representation in both the Old Testament and Freud's psychoanalytic framework. This impossible element transcends gender, as in Séverin's case, residing at the core of the *Nebenmensch* and potentially attaching itself to the maternal object or any object couching the question of desire from an early stage. It represents the boundless and terrifying backstage of existence itself. Perhaps unsurprisingly, the foreclosure of the paternal signifier disrupts the order and appeasement it traditionally provides. This, in turn, brings to scene the Symbolic impasse that embodies the Real, pushing it beyond the frame of meaning and into the realm of the unsymbolizable.

Notes

1 Supplementary device, which is a translation of the French word *suppléance*, comes from the verb *suppléer*. meaning to replace or substitute something when it's lacking or faulty. It's a concept that Lacan develops in his topology of the Borromean knot, more precisely in Seminar 22, *R.S.I.*, when he mentions the need for a fourth loop to be created and connected in a certain manner so as to impede the detachment of the three loops or the three registers. This fourth loop is for the neurotic the NotF, which is foreclosed in psychosis.

2 According to E. Pluth (2007), a portion of jouissance remains elusive within the fantasmatic framework, beyond the grasp of the fundamental fantasy. Not all jouissance and the Other's desire can be fully apprehended by this fundamental fantasy. "In fantasy, the subject is not put into a relation with this part of jouissance that does not get 'written' in the fantasy. For this reason, the fantasy is indeed something like a window on the [R]eal. It permits access to the [R]eal under controlled conditions, conditions that effectively protect us from the [R]eal, while allowing access to a colonized, tamed [R]eal" (Pluth, 2007, pp. 87–88). Later, Pluth states that the "fantasy not only joins the child to the Other (a junction that serves to give a place to the subject in the Other, and also serves to sustain a signification for jouissance), but it also presupposes and preserves a disjunction and an expulsion from the Other and 'being'" (Pluth, 2007, p. 94). I remind

the reader of Russell's paradox of the Language set {A}, introduced in Chapter 2, where every speaking being is trapped. Perhaps Lacanian theorization of jouissance and fundamental fantasy offers a glimpse into this Symbolic impasse and the Real where the subject finds itself. Being joined and disjoined, alienated and separated from the Other, seems a structural necessity, a metaphysical priority to become a human subject and pose a framework to the excesses of the Thing.

3 Other jouissance, a jouissance not-all, is a form of satisfaction that comes from the female side, $\overline{\forall x}\, \Phi x$, from the Other (God). When a speaking subject positions itself as not-all within the phallic function, it takes the female side (Lacan, 1972–1973, p. 72). Being on the side of Woman means being partly excluded from phallic jouissance. Being not-all implies that Woman has a supplementary jouissance beyond the phallus, which skims the Real. This is Other jouissance, a jouissance not-all, an ineffable experience of jouissance. Probably the figure of the mystic's ecstasy, like St. Theresa of Avila's transverberation, are the most common approximations to this type of jouissance.

4 Matheme is an expression used by Lacan since 1968 to name the algebraic-type formulae composed of symbols whose configuration tries to expound the way the unconscious operates. The purpose of the use of mathematical writing and schemas is to propose an alternative to speech and verbal language, to the Imaginary and the Symbolic. For Lacan it is the closest formalization to grasp the Real.

13

Dealing with psychosis and discourse

A case study

13.1. The non-extraction of object a

In Lacan's discourses, any of the four components can occupy one of four positions. In Seminar *The Other Side of Psychoanalysis*, he introduced two different terms in two distinct positions of the discourses that do not appear in the final version of Seminar *Le savoir du psychanalyste*, lecture of February 3, 1972. Instead of production, Lacan writes loss, and instead of the agent, he writes desire (Lacan, 1969–1970, p. 93). In each of the five discourses, he identifies a loss in which one of the four elements can be found. The Master's and Capitalist's discourses both place object *a* in the locus of loss/production. Any Postmodern individual can situate itself in either of these two discourses, and it is impossible to fully escape them; our subjective positions will inevitably lean on them both. Thus, we are producers of the system, supposed masters of ourselves, embodying a value, a workforce, a job, a citizen with rights and duties, hence, a deontic subject. At the same time, we suffer some kind of loss, sacrifice, submission, or relinquishment that the Master demands of us. However, the individual has a margin of maneuver. It can rely more on the contestation or questioning of power, putting knowledge in the place of production/loss and in the locus of truth the object cause of desire (Hysteric's discourse). Or, it can produce a new master signifier and in the locus of truth leave a new knowledge about the symptom (Analyst's discourse). These alternatives are not offered to everybody though, and we mostly succumb to the Master's or Capitalist's discourse.

What happens to the psychotic, who is outside of discourse? If we start from the lack of lack (¬S(Ⱥ)) that the non-extraction of object *a* implies, this *plus-de-jouir* cannot be located in any of the positions allowed by the Lacanian algebra of discourses, or at least it is problematic for the psychotic. In a lecture to psychiatrists, *Petit discours aux psychiatres* (1967), Lacan alludes to where this object might be found for the mad man: he "has his cause in his pocket; that's why he's mad". He is referring to object petit *a*, the cause of desire. The non-extraction of this object has consequences for the psychotic. Its extraction leads to the formation of the framework of reality given by fundamental fantasy (Lacan, 1959, p. 487). This fantasy ($ ◊ *a*) orients the subject's desire and limits their possibilities of action. It favors

DOI: 10.4324/9781032663616-17

a projection of object *a* onto the Other, acting as a reference point and creating a boundary to an infinite drift.

> [T]he consequence [of the extraction of object *a*] is that the choice of the subject manifests itself, in its way of positioning itself in the face of lack… the father, a wife, a job, a hobby, a lobby, writing, the psychoanalyst, the search for the Truth, etc. […] Absences obeying the structure, that of language: of the sexual relation, of a signifier in the Other, of Woman, of metalanguage, all declared, one after the other, that they are not.
>
> (Braunstein, 2017, p. 54)

A published case study can illustrate how to read psychosis from the non-extraction of object *a* and the subject's negotiation of discourse within the Master's ordinance, master of himself. This discourse places the subject, knowledge, the master signifier, and *plus-de-jouir* in different positions. The case is about a man who has been performing non-mainstream body modifications for many years, all geared towards a project he calls "alien cyborg". His objective is to physically become this, and he does this through extreme mutilations, implants, tattoos, and body performances. He has never manifested hallucinations, a persecutory or paranoid position, or any type of negative symptom, and he has never sought psychological or psychiatric consultation (Londoño, Gil, and Marín, 2023). However, I will show how he is still situated outside of discourse and how he manages to sort out a psychotic structure.

13.2. A case of nonmainstream body modifications

Mr. Z is a 26-year-old man who is found amid an investigation in the university context about body modifications and their relationship with symptomatic and psychosomatic experiences. The term "psychosomatic" refers to the combination of linear and permanent relationships between mental processes and their corresponding somatic responses, which include not only somatoform disorders or somatizations (conversion symptoms). Within the psychosomatic spectrum, close to what it is currently known as Body Integrity Identity Disorder, there is room for all manifestations where the subjective experience of the body generates problems and discomfort for the subject at an emotional, affective, and personal level, such as transgenderism or gender dysphoria, cases of psychotic patients and hypochondria, subjects with body image disorders, bulimia and anorexia, chronic pain, or functional disorders, among others. Medicine and biology have tried to rescue people from the impasse of psychosomatic manifestations, especially those in psychiatric populations. Medical scientists have sought to explain the origin of these conditions/symptoms through biological, pathophysiological, neurocognitive, and even genetic abnormalities and dysfunctions. However, their explanatory proposals seem unable to fully explain the intertwining of the mind/body relation. That which speaks or says something in and through the body is precisely what cannot be signified, that is, what we cannot put into signifiers, words, and, of course, make sense of it or determine a position with respect to S_2 and *a*: it is outside of discourse! However, it is not my intention to turn these psychosomatic manifestations into some sort of nosological entity or some new brand of disorders. It is a way of describing a series of phenomena that many subjects live and experience concerning their relationship with their own body image and esthesias, and which can be disturbing.

Now, we encounter the symptoms and discomforts that do not speak but are written down or leave a trace of their passage across the body. Unlike conversion hysteria other psychosomatic ailments are directly connected to jouissance and the Real. They are connected to a way of living and experiencing the body and can serve as a support to stabilize and compensate for (*suppléer*) certain psychiatric pathologies (Castanet, 2017; Lacan, 1975–1976). Body art may be used as a supplementary device to self-heal and stabilize from certain types of psychological distress, not only in psychiatric populations but also outside of hospitals and psychological services. This can help us understand the role of body art in mental health.

This population is not commonly applicant for psychotherapy and even fewer for psychoanalytic consultation, so approaching them is not easy and requires going out to search for them in order to interview and get to know about their experiences. Precisely the self-treatment and the direct work on their body make them not usually applicants for psychoanalysis. Many of them become famous in social networks, and tend to make public their own transformations and life history.

Mr. Z was left at an early age in the care of his maternal grandmother by his mother, who abandoned him with her at birth and moved to another country. The father was murdered in strange circumstances shortly before he was born, and Mr. Z does not seem at all interested in his father or his life story; for him, it is something that has already happened, and he does not remember much. He is also not curious about what the paternal story is or who his father was. Similarly, there is little that he knows about his mother, who did not really watch over him or take care of his upbringing. With his grandmother, he comments that the relationship was always cold and distant; they never got along. She died when he was 15 years old, and since then he has lived alone and managed to support himself financially with small jobs. There are few or no childhood memories, which he doesn't seem to want to talk about or at least feel interested in talking about. Those memories are simply gone, or they *don't count anymore.*

He began body modifications at the age of 10, with empirical face piercings, which means that he himself performed these procedures, having at a certain moment more than 30 facial piercings. After his grandmother's death, the subject began his process of extreme body modifications; he designed a project, naming it "alien-cyborg" based on what the subject considered appropriate for his appearance, in this case, something that had never seen, an "alien-type robot", where Hans Ruedi Giger is the author of reference.

The subject usually practices body suspension with the intention of inflicting pain on himself. He claims that "*the taste for body hook suspension was born from my pleasure to see how much my body could bear because I remember that since*

I was, I don't know, about 8 years old, looking for ways of inflicting pain". His extreme modifications started with scarifications on the back. Scarifications are procedures in which deep incisions or etchings are made to the skin, which leave large scabs and scars, thus generating a figure or shape on the skin.

At the age of 17, the project began to take its course, beginning with the first modification in which the nipples and the navel were mutilated with a scalpel, he then proceeded to remove first the whole nail from a finger of the right hand, then later the upper phalanx of the same finger. Later subdermal implants were introduced in both arms and penis, his eyes (the sclera) were tattooed in deep black, and days later most of his ears were amputated, then he proceeded to tattoo most of his face in black with asymmetric designs. After tattooing his face, the first modifications were made to his lips, which were based first on the excision of part of the lower lip and bifurcation of the upper one. Right after this procedure, he lengthened his nostrils; this operation was based on amputating part of the skin tissue over the nasal cavity and then performing a "stretching" or "lengthening". After a few years, the subject decided to remove the subdermal implants from the penis and arms, then he excised one of his testicles all by himself. All these procedures were performed without any anesthesia and almost all were performed by him. It should be noted that in addition to these procedures, the subject practices body, facial, and genital hook suspensions, where in genital suspension he stages testicular weight-lifting and genital torture in public spectacles. Finally, the next procedure that the subject has in mind for his project is to remove the penis, but before removing the organ, he wants to perform bifurcation and subdermal implants in it. He also aims to tattoo his entire body in black, a procedure better known as "blackout" and to get a tattoo that traces a red line around the edge of the body (Londoño, Gil, and Marín, 2023).

The subject reports no history of psychology or psychiatry treatment, episodes of anxiety or depression, hallucinatory experiences, language disorders, persecutory or paranoid ideas, or sleep or eating disorders. Affective lability, abulia, and flat affect were also ruled out. Even his goal of becoming an alien-cyborg could be ruled out as delusional because it aligns with the (hyper)modern discourse of self-creation, individual life projects, and the right to self-determination. He reports having been married and fathering a child as a result of that relationship, but he soon separated from his partner because he was not interested in relationships, let alone sexual relationships. He is not interested in knowing about or being committed to others, and sexuality does not interest him either.

13.3. Reading the case through the Capitalist's discourse

According to current taxonomies, such as the DSM, Mr. Z could be classified with schizoid personality disorder due to his lack of interest in sexual relations or close relationships with others, and perhaps also body dysmorphic disorder due to his preoccupation with his perceived defects. However, these defects are not the same as those typically considered in the DSM. For example, Mr. Z does not consider himself abnormal, ugly, or deformed; on the contrary, he believes himself to be *too normal*. This is the precise issue. Additionally, Mr. Z does not meet any of the other criteria for body dysmorphic disorder. One could also consider the diagnosis of nonsuicidal self-injury in the chapter of "Conditions for Further Study". However, Mr. Z's behaviors do not cause him distress, and to a certain extent they are socially sanctioned (e.g., tattoos, piercings) (APA, 2013). There has been recent discussion about a diagnosis known as Body Integrity Identity Disorder, yet it's not officially acknowledged in the DSM and lacks legal recognition. Perhaps, Disorders of Bodily Distress and Bodily Experience (6C20) in the ICD-11 could account for someone like Mr. Z, but still the criteria don't really apply to him either.

Apart from that, it is difficult to know where to classify this subject. The idea of pointing to a structural diagnosis can be fruitful, especially when psychosis appears so veiled and out of reach of the classical way of dealing with diagnosis in the current psychiatric tradition. He could even pass as a subject without any diagnosis, especially since he is not a seeker of medical-psychological consultation nor does he seem to be in a state of distress or emergency, or at least he does not imply that he is in that situation. It is because of the eccentricity of his purpose and the unusualness of his actions that he appears to be quite counterintuitive, even disconcerting to the Other. What is striking for the Other is precisely the extent of his intention—the point to which he feels capable of reaching in order to achieve an ego-ideal that seems impossible, physically impossible—that runs up against an insurmountable wall that Mr. Z doesn't seem to want to contemplate. The Real for this subject is not an obstacle; he can move forward, and nothing seems to stop him. The fact that there is no alarm or SOS signal to the Other, as Schreber could have requested when he found himself cornered by a threatening Other jouissance, indicates that at the moment there is no Other that could be attributed with a knowledge (lack of *point de capiton*) able to ballast the drifting body experience. The closest thing to knowledge is a condensed and semi-legalized jouissance that wraps the "alien-cyborg project".

Up until here, one could suppose an outside-discourse of his entire purpose, cutting him off from the social bond. Mr. Z is in a position of absolute mastery of himself; he believes he is in full control of his body, of which he supposes possessing a flawless knowledge; nothing can leak out of this expertise of the limits of the body and how far the scalpel can go. Those who listen to him cannot legitimize or make what he says count as an acceptable social fact. In this sense, his behavior seems deinstitutionalized and he presents himself as something that does not count-as-one, an odd multiple narrative, or his counting is problematic for the elements that may belong to the {A}, especially when the whole purpose collides with the Real. This is even less when it is observed that what sustains the project cannot be historicized; it is outside of any historicization.

What does this eventful site of performances and self-mutilations mask to the Other? The past and the symbolic consistency of his "alien-cyborg" project do not have significant support within an elaborate, conscientious plan, legalized under the Father's law, and that favors the social bond. It seems more like a desire to build a body around something where desire can be focused on an activity seen as appreciable, acceptable by the contemporary Master's discourses (body art), and which gives the subject the possibility of treating his jouissance and allowing cohesion to his image; in this effort, he maintains a semblance of social bond.

As $, Mr Z is made, he becomes a subject; although he does not hint at a division, his project, and the indelible image of transformation into a creature out of this world, demonstrate his potential to make a One, to become a subset of {A}, a subject semblance. He introduces an S_1 where there wasn't one, and he *intervenes* by starting to count from the moment he gives himself a new identity and a new name. One could argue that his history begins the moment he enters within this decision to step into a new body and name himself as a new species. A species-as-operator, naming an inconsistent multiple, founding a self-made NotF.

There is a semblance of an eventful project that grants a means of stabilization but that can collapse in the face of any medical complication. The project seeks to rewrite the history of Mr. Z and reinstate him in a position in which he can maintain a social bond, hence his tours in the country to carry out shows of genital torture and hook suspensions, and his multiple appearances on television and on social networks, etc. He turned into an object of curiosity that holds a place in the bond grounded on the Other's gaze and morbidity. If he holds on to something, it is from the new nomination that the rejection of the NotF did not allow to carry out in him; calling himself an alien-cyborg awards him that which his own name and surname did not accord him from a father who was not there and without history, and a mother who did not name him or care for him, who did not count in the process of naming and negation. In this, Mr. Z is a self-made man or self-made hybrid, and if anyone embodies that motto of (post) modernity it is he.

> *Well, the project is then, as I was telling you... I wanted to do a body modification project because I didn't want to... just start doing things and I wanted to take everything down a path to be able to self-denominate or call myself something else, so I looked for... or I was thinking about how I wanted to see myself, what I wanted to do and that's when the idea of an alien cyborg was born.*

First, he wanted to just be a machine, but it looked too banal. Afterward, he discovered Giger's aliens, and he wanted a merger of both ideas:

> *...then I began to see how I could unite both things until I reached a point where I said "well I am going to be a kind of alien cyborg, an alien machine"... and I can take them through my own path to give/see if I can find a way to unite... those two tendencies in my body.*
>
> (Londoño, Gil, and Marin, 2023, p. 8)

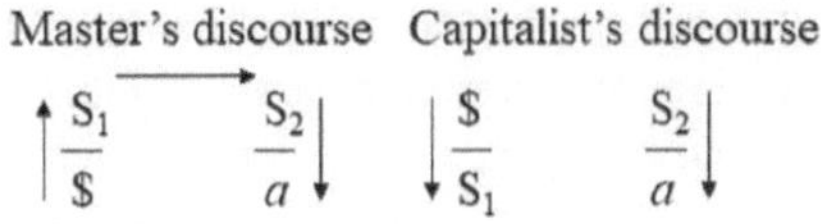

Figure 13.1

Here, it is no longer just the place of master of himself that he occupies within this discourse of the Master; Mr. Z flows in an apparent social bond, not as the classic master but as the modern master of himself. That is to say, he finds himself squarely posited in the Capitalist's discourse.

Here, I point out that the Capitalist's discourse has a couple of changes concerning the classical Master's discourse.

As shown in Figure 11.1, the Capitalist's discourse not only inverts the elements in the place of the agent and of the truth, but also removes the upper arrow that goes from the agent (the one who acts or is acted upon) to the other. Additionally, on the agent's side, the subject acts on the truth of S_1. This means that the Capitalist's discourse hardly creates a social bond; it is a limitless discourse, as indicated by the absence of the upper arrow, which means that "there is no impossibility" (Lacan, 1972–1973, p. 16). The $ is in the place of the consumer and consumption; the objects of consumption are addressed to this consumer, but Mr. Z himself is the place and object of consumption. Knowledge is on the side of a pseudoscience or pseudotechnique that he believes he possesses about the body (S_2) by being a bricoleur of it. His body is a fetish, merchandise, spectacle, and space for experimentation with pseudo-technical knowledge; he offers it as a commodity to the gaze and as jouissance in the void. That is to say, it is not a shared jouissance that condescends to desire and to the Other but which presents as a mere parade to the gaze. Unlimited jouissance and the foreclosure of castration (which does not make the foreclosed disappear but rather reappear in the Real) are the leitmotifs of the Capitalist's discourse, where an imperative of jouissance and the injunction "anything is possible" predominate.

If there is castration, it must go through him but not through the Symbolic and Imaginary registers; castration did not previously operate on him. He is the active and patient voice of the extraction of object *a*, an object that returns in the Real in the form of a body in excess, where the lack is lacking, $\neg S(\not{A})$. Shards of *plus-de-jouir* not legalized by the NotF generate deregulated jouissance and provoke a desire for transformation, for a life project, pushing him to literally extract it from his body. Here lies the paradox, the ambivalence of the attempt to make an event in Mr. Z of the project, to tell a story and be able to name it, to turn it into a subset that counts within that great set of Language {A} and that of myths. This favors the fact that Mr. Z can more or less sustain himself in existence and this has not led him to decompensation or a psychic outburst.

There does not seem to have been an individual myth in Mr. Z that tells how he was able to solve the impasse of maternal desire and jouissance (or, in this case, that of the grandmother). The emergence of his first instinctual experiences in what could have been the care and attention of his grandmother as a maternal object did not cause the implementation of castration, of a myth of castration, loss, and the phobic reaction together with its consecutive resolution within that myth. No one seemed to intercede on that point, as Hans's father could have done at the given moment, even if he did so at the request of Freud himself (Lacan, 1956–1957, pp. 271–273). The intercession of a third element, as an instance present or referred to in the speech, produces effects in the Imaginary rearrangement of distressing elements of the Oedipal relationship and favors the symbolic exchange, the separation of the drive object, so that what appears as voracious in the image of the Other caregiver loses its crushing force.

Mr. Z must directly write the unique and decisive myth over his body. On the other hand, there is no narrated family or paternal myth on which it can be based; there is no family romance fantasy in which he can tell a story of his origins, lineage, and affiliation. There were no points of reference or support for the assumption of his image and his identity; the peer was not a point of comparison, the image of the other being "*too common*" for him. What society considers "normal" holds no sway for him. It's outside his current understanding, defined not by fixed images but by the ongoing process of his transformation. His path to "normalcy", then, lies not in conformity but in fulfilling this transformative project, becoming who he is meant to be. The reflection in the mirror holds no familiar spark, no sense of self shared with another.

Mr. Z's pursuit of stabilization seems primarily driven by his focus on the Real body and his struggles with jouissance. He views the removal of the object, the source of his drifting image and excess jouissance, as the only potential solution. However, the self-therapeutic process itself seems only to offer temporary relief. While self-mutilation aims to weigh down the overwhelming anxiety and jouissance, its effect appears fleeting. Regardless of the risks, Mr. Z feels compelled to continue this painful project, driven by the desperate hope of achieving that elusive stability.

Mr. Z's experience of bodily jouissance hinges on the extreme swings between pain and pleasure, a relentless push-pull that inscribes its mark on him. This endless loop fuels the delusion of his body as a perfect machine, a vessel capable of withstanding any imaginable assault, injury, or pressure. He operates under the unshakeable belief that his body is impervious to limits.

Conclusion

For Lacan, the father is nothing more than a reference (Lacan, 1971, p. 173). He is castrated, to the point of being nothing more than a number (Lacan, 1971, p. 174). Lacan suggests that the saga of the kings of a nation indicates that the number serves to classify and identify each of the persons who received the same name and were crowned. However, Lacan sees the number more as the term *nombre* in French, that is, within an ordinality of natural numbers. As I indicated in Chapter 1, the count must start at 0, that is, there would be a starting point, a Father with a value of 0, an inexistent father which sets necessity. However, the Name of God enters in cardinality, as something exterior to the system it inaugurates (Reinhard and Reinhard Lupton, 2003). It is from this point that Freud places the origin Father in the myth of the parricide of the primal horde (Freud, 1913, pp. 141–144) and, similarly, from this point that Lacan places it in the dialogue of Moses with the burning bush when Yahwe reveals his name. When Lacan supports these events, he is not assuming that they actually happened. He is not saying that the parricide of the primal horde or the fact that Moses heard the name of God were actual events that took place at a specific time and place in history. Perhaps it is the accumulation of events of all kinds, correlatable within a long historical process, that favored the creation of these myths. The origin and creation myths respond to a necessity, a necessity that is generated only by speaking beings and the structural lack of language. It is not something that is reduced to or ends up crystallizing into something biological or even phylogenetic. The necessity is not "produced" or put into words; it is something that is assumed, inexistent, and arises retroactively as a result of the activity of thought. This is, necessity only becomes necessity because we are doomed to think and speak.

> Inexistence is only produced in retroaction [*après-coup*] from which there first arises necessity, namely from a discourse in which it manifests itself prior to the logician reaching it himself as a second consequence, that is, at the same time that inexistence itself. Its end is to be reduced right where this necessity manifests itself, prior to him.
>
> (Lacan, 1971–1972, p. 41)

This is, the number nought and inexistence arise *post hoc*, in retroaction, after the logician Frege and his predecessors came to postulate them. The number nought appears as a logical necessity, as it cannot be identical with itself. For it to be so, it has to give way to the count; in this case, the step toward 1. One implies repeating it for all things in the world that count as one, and which acquire their own name, becoming the unit of the natural number.

> In order for the number to pass from the repetition of the 1 of the identical to that of its ordered succession, in order for the logical dimension to gain its autonomy definitively, without any reference to the real the zero has to appear [...].
>
> In this engendering of the zero, I have stressed that it is supported by the proposition that truth is. If no object falls under the concept of non-identical-with-itself, it is because truth must be saved. If there are no things which are not identical to themselves, it is because non-identity with itself is contradictory to the very dimension of truth. To its concept, we assign the zero.
>
> It is this decisive proposition that *the concept of not-identical-with-itself is assigned by the number zero* which sutures logical discourse.
>
> (Miller, 1977, p. 5)

This 0-value suture that Miller refers to indicates that that is a logical necessity to organize truth—the locus of what cannot present itself. In this inexistence, the logical movement of speaking beings is to begin to count and institute ordinality; the origin myth has this function. That logical movement is also metaphysical, namely, the a priori principles of thought in Aristotle's *Metaphysics* (identity, non-contradiction, and the law of the excluded middle), necessity of a first cause (unmoved mover), and modality (the necessary and the contingent, the possible and the impossible). There must be a cause for something to be, something out of which a thing comes to be and persists (material cause), is the essence and form (formal cause), acts as a primary source of change (efficient cause), or has a purpose (final cause). In his *Metaphysics*, Aristotle says that there is not only a cause but a first cause for everything that happens. If everything has a cause, there must be something that is the cause of everything. There should be a first engine that sets everything in motion, a principle, and a first cause for an action or a movement. For something to be as it is, it must come from something that caused it (Aristotle, 1952a). The metaphysical support is a priori to any possible first cause; it is retroactive in that it seeks to describe what a cause is and how it is based on what the set of signifiers in the context in which we are ingrained has outlined for us about the modalities and the first causes. That which is presented appears as *a multiple* that is, that can turn into one, and its counting causes effects in the world. The subject attributes causality not just by empirical observation but by counting a set of multiples as such, as cause, by the intervention in the eventful site. The need to ascribe causality to any experienced phenomenon drives the subject to make use of myth to cover any metaphysical gap. Especially, to the questions "where do we come from?", "how did we get here?", "how do we get our place in a family?" And these causal questions can move us to consequential ones or final causes like "what is our purpose in life?" or "what is the meaning of life?"

The knotting of the three registers—the Real, the Symbolic, and the Imaginary—guarantees the apprehension of reality through counting, naming, and re-presenting, covering the gap and the Thing that sits in the void. However, as Badiou reminds us, the structure or the count-as-one alone is not enough to avoid fixing the void in a presentation, which would lead to its depletion. "The fundamental reason behind this insufficiency is that something, within presentation, escapes the count: this something is nothing other than the count itself" (Badiou, 2005, p. 93). So, for there to be no emergence of the void in a presentation, the structure must remain structured; that is, the metastructure must operate. This metastructure is what the first body of the signifier, its first adumbration, will serve to name. Now, this possibility should not be taken for granted as an innate development of the speaking being, but requires an encounter with the Other under its voice and care, by its introduction to the world of the signifier and discourse. In this encounter, the first form of dialectic is established in the early judicative movements in the act of naming and apprehending presentations. That is, in the production of attribution and judgments of existence, or how to start employing the signifier. Hence, any action that is accompanied by the first forms of negation and naming as a suture-to-being makes any presentation to begin to count-as-one. Negating and naming suppose the suture of the nought in its functioning since only that which is identical with itself can be named and exist. It is crucial to ensure that each element is accounted for within the chain of signifiers, specifically within the register of the Symbolic. Otherwise, a signifier may remain uncounted, leading to its reappearance in the Real, manifesting as psychotic hallucination, delusion, or the compulsive repetition of an indelible image, impossible to subjetivicize—or the reduction of the body to a mere object lacking a master-signifier for consistency. In essence, any displayed action with symbolic and existential value, when there is no NotF on its horizon, will resurface in the Real, exposing the distress of the Thing.

Now, the myth of the origins and foundations of the Western world passed through Judeo-Christianity, settling in the books of the Old Testament, which in turn came from the myths of previous Mesopotamian civilizations. The *Enuma Elish* or the books of the Pentateuch assure the origin myths of past peoples but insist on the present day, as an unconscious frame, on the functioning of the social group, and where truth is invested; truth around which the world of speech is organized, where we move from chaos to an order in which the world's inhabitants can inhabit. That is, following some precepts, a set of visions, of customs and practices that are justified within myths. Language both feeds on and participates in the assemblage of these myths. It also suffers from myth, and in that circularity of mutual influence, myth traces an impossible, where truth lies somewhere between contradictory and identical points (Lacan, 1969–1970, pp. 126–127). Strictly speaking, they outline the relationship of nought with one, and of what is different and identical at the same time. For instance, if one takes into account Frege's passage in §77 of his *Grundlagen*, he states that "1 is the Number which belongs to the concept 'identical with 0'... 1 follows in the series of natural numbers directly after 0" (Frege, 1960, §77). A few lines later, he indicates, "it is perhaps worth pointing out that our definition of the number 1 does not presuppose, for its objective legitimacy, any matter of observed fact" (Frege, 1960, §77). The number 1 belongs to the set of numbers "identical with 0", identical in the sense that in such a set there is at least *one* object that falls into it, 0. Nought, as such, named, uttered, or written, turns into something that can be counted-as-one, this is, precisely when it is named, uttered, or written. This is just the logical movement of presentation that creation myths seek to re-present. At this point, God, or any interweaving of deities, emerges *ex nihilo* as the first or master-signifier (S_1), or the one to whom we attribute the starting point of creation, *i.e.*, from chaos to order, from void to name. The signifier of God is *the* element of the set "identical with 0"; as it were, how from the {ø} one starts counting. This passage puts in tension the dichotomy of being and non-being, identity and non-identity.

In this context, Lacan introduces his conceptual proposal of the NotF. Here, like a father, God is assigned the function of creation. The question of origins and creation, which is formulated to humanity as it is to any child, leads from the father who conceives the individual to the father who conceives the universe. The mother lost her place in this mythology, not simply because of patriarchal bias and oppression, but because maternity does not typically generate as many questions and uncertainty. A woman can rarely hide or deny her pregnancy and labor; the mother's identity is not as frequently questioned as the father's. Being a father is confusing in terms of his functions, his role, and even his need for conceiving a child. For instance, in today's world, in vitro fertilization and single parenthood demonstrate that a father is not necessary for conception or for creating a family (Lacan, 1955–1956, pp. 292–293; Eidelsztein, 2019).

Now, the concept of NotF has always been associated in the Lacanian psychoanalytic milieu with psychosis; it has become almost a term that metonymically leads to the idea of what psychosis is and its etiology. However, it is not always so obvious to be able to see how this signifier is missing or did not operate in a specific case. Much less how the phenomena of psychosis are observed outside of non-Judeo-Christian cultures where that signifier would not circulate, or would but in a different guise (see the case of West Africa, in Ortigues and Ortigues, 1984). Lacan said that, for instance, the Oedipus complex was for the Sudanese "just rather a thin joke", a "tiny detail within an immense myth" (Lacan, 1953–1954, p. 86). This is not only an ethnopsychiatric matter, but it is important to bear in mind that its configuration occurs in a context that responds to a certain tradition and genealogy, which I sought to outline in Part 2 of the book, but that cannot be extrapolated to all latitudes.

In this, the predominance of a discursive organization of subjectivities inside the social bond is key to understanding how an individual stands with regard to jouissance, knowledge, and the master-signifiers of an epoch and context. How discourse is organized is not only about the relationship of the agent/semblance with its production, supported by truth; it is also about the circulation of signifiers within this Klein four-group of discourse that Lacan sought to formalize. And the signifiers are organized, oriented, and chained in a certain way that favors not only the production of meaning but also the fashion in which meaning is produced and the use one ascribes to it within the libidinal economy (in the dialectic of pleasure-unpleasure), and desire. The NotF fulfills this paradoxical ordering role of the employment of the signifier, by being its first structure, while being at the same time a signifier of the Law, "a term that maintains the basic system of words at a certain distance or relational dimension. Something is missing and his [the psychotic] real effort at substitution and 'significization' is directed in desperation at that" (Lacan, 1959–1960, p. 66). As a button tie (*point de capiton*), one can observe how psychosis exemplifies the way in which this function is uncoordinated, failing, which does not imply that the subject may be incapable of speaking or enunciating a purpose, but there is nothing that can ballast its purposes definitely, or that could organize them, providing a place to lack and closure. Even tying up desire and law seems conflictive in certain cases as we saw with Jim Jones or Deutsch's case. This is not limited to an immediate or short-term purpose, it also implies long-term intentions and purposes, which include long-term and lasting bonds with the Other. This is why it is so frequent that many stabilized psychotics tend to abandon their jobs, their relationships, or any life project very easily to start some new one that will turn out to be just as slight and frail. Nonetheless, on the opposite side, the button tie can freeze in a signifier (holophrase) that substitutes the NotF, serving as a supplementary device but petrifying meaning over an absolute object and generating a strong psychic dependence on it. The subject hooks onto a signifier that turns into a life guarantor but impedes *aphanisis*. This was the case with Mr. Z, who was unable to respond when asked about the hypothetical impossibility of him being able to perform the "surgical" procedures necessary for his life project, claiming that the idea was inconceivable to him. This suggests that without his transformation project, he would likely have fallen into a psychotic crisis requiring some third-party intervention.

Now, how does a mythical entity that has effects on the ordering of the collective operate on an individual? This question becomes more relevant after the profound mutation that Modernity has entailed in the West. Let us remember that Modernity repositions the individual as the center of the discourse towards which the master-signifiers converge, but it is also the starting point of initiatives around which the meaning of the purposes and the ultimate goals of existence turn. Modernity opened the gate into the abyss of meaning and the Real, and committed each subject directly to having to locate its referents of desire and ego-ideal, precisely as a superegoic demand. Being the owner of oneself and judge of one's actions means that each one must build one's *individual myth*. What is this myth built on? On what the desire of the mother and the NotF, together with the predominant discourse, draw as the limit of the possible while encompassing some narrative about the impossible. In this, the neurotic has at its disposal a small arsenal to assemble its own symptom and myth, as in the case of Lanzer, the Rat Man, or little Hans.

While Schreber, Aimée or Mr. Z, when confronted with the question of the Father signifier, purpose, and their origins reflect a void of meaning, a ruin of presentation, the open rift reveals the Thing in its most penetrating inexistence. Faced with these phenomena of perplexity, depersonalization-derealization, cenesthopathies, and lack of response, unchaining of the signifier and jouissance, the psychotic must then have recourse to a massive movement of the signifier, either through a delusional metaphor or through direct treatment of jouissance in the body. This is seen both in Schreber and in Mr. Z, whose overture to the Thing is, in its first instance, framed in an indelible image and stated in a proposition, *i.e.*, a proto-fundamental fantasy that contains a distressing and unframed jouissance. The advantage is that the psychotic can set into motion a work on the body and the signifier facilitating the re-inscription of the one of the presentation, offering a certain consistency, although the indelible image permeates every presentation, which means that the psychotic must constantly deal with a surplus of unregulated jouissance. However, the psychotic subject also has the clues to begin a self-healing process; he has keys to guide him towards the possibility of a more or less lasting stabilization.

References of J. Lacan's works

Lacan, J. (1931). Structures des psychoses paranoïaques. *Semaine des hôpitaux de Paris, 14*, pp. 437–445.

Lacan, J. (1932). *De la psychose paranoïaque dans ses rapports avec la personnalité*. Paris: Éditions du Seuil (Points poche), 1975.

Lacan, J. (1938). Les complexes familiaux dans la formation de l'individu. In *Autres écrits*. Paris: Éditions du Seuil, 2001.

Lacan, J. (1946). Presentation on psychical causality. In Écrits, *The First Complete Edition in English*. Trans. B. Fink. New York: W.W. Norton & Co., 2006.

Lacan, J. (1949). The mirror stage as formative of the *I* function as revealed in psychoanalytic experience. In Écrits, *The First Complete Edition in English*. Trans. B. Fink. New York: W.W. Norton & Co., 2006.

Lacan, J. (1950). A theoretical introduction to the functions of psychoanalysis in criminology. In Écrits, *The First Complete Edition in English*. Trans. B. Fink. New York: W.W. Norton & Co., 2006.

Lacan, J. (1953). The neurotic's individual myth. *The Psychoanalytic Quarterly, 48*(3), 405–425, 1979. Doi: 10.1080/21674086.1979.11926884.

Lacan, J. (1953a). The function and field of speech and language in psychoanalysis. In Écrits, *The First Complete Edition in English*. Trans. B. Fink. New York: W.W. Norton & Co., 2006.

Lacan, J. (1953–1954). *The Seminar of Jacques Lacan, book I. Freud's Papers on Technique*. Trans. J. Forrester. New York: W.W. Norton & Co., 1991.

Lacan, J. (1954). Response to Jean Hyppolite's commentary on Freud's "Verneinung". In Écrits, *The First Complete Edition in English*. Trans. B. Fink. New York: W.W. Norton & Co., 2006.

Lacan, J. (1954–1955). *The Seminar of Jacques Lacan, book II. The Ego in Freud's Theory and in the Technique of Psychoanalysis*. Trans. S. Tomaselli. New York: W.W. Norton & Co., 1991.

Lacan, J. (1955–1956). *The Seminar of Jacques Lacan, book III. The Psychoses*. Trans. R. Grigg. New York: W.W. Norton & Co., 1993.

Lacan, J., Lévi-Strauss, C., Paulme, D., Diopp, M.M., Dumont, L., Wahl, J., Merleau-Ponty, M., Leiris, Métraux, M., Tubiana, M., and Goldmann, L. (1956). *Sur les rapports entre la mythologie et le rituel*. Société Française de Philosophie. Retrieved from: https://www.sofrphilo.fr/activites-scientifiques-de-la-sfp/conferences/grandes-conferences-en-telechargement/

Lacan, J. (1956–1957). *The Seminar of Jacques Lacan, book IV. The Object Relation*. Trans. A.R. Price. Cambridge: Polity Press, 2020.

Lacan, J. (1957). The instance of the letter in the unconscious, or reason since Freud. In Écrits, *The First Complete Edition in English*. Trans. B. Fink. New York: W.W. Norton & Co., 2006.

Lacan, J. (1957–1958). *The Seminar of Jacques Lacan, book V. Formations of the Unconscious*. Trans. R. Grigg. Cambridge: Polity Press, 2017.

Lacan, J. (1958). The signification of the phallus. In Écrits, *The First Complete Edition in English*. Trans. B. Fink. New York: W.W. Norton & Co., 2006.

Lacan, J. (1958a). The direction of the treatment and the principles of its powers. In Écrits, *The First Complete Edition in English*. Trans. B. Fink. New York: W.W. Norton & Co., 2006.

Lacan, J. (1958–1959). *The Seminar of Jacques Lacan, book VI. Desire and Its Interpretation*. Trans. B. Fink. Cambridge: Polity Press, 2019.

Lacan, J. (1959). On a question prior to any possible treatment of psychosis. In Écrits, *The First Complete Edition in English*. Trans. B. Fink. New York: W.W. Norton & Co., 2006.

Lacan, J. (1959–1960). *The Seminar of Jacques Lacan, book VII. The Ethics of Psychoanalysis*. Trans. D. Porter. New York: W.W. Norton & Co., 1992.

Lacan, J. (1960). The subversion of the subject and the dialectic of desire in Freudian unconscious. In Écrits, *The First Complete Edition in English*. Trans. B. Fink. New York: W.W. Norton & Co., 2006.

Lacan, J. (1960a). Remarks on Daniel Lagache's presentation: "Psychoanalysis and personality structure". In Écrits, *The First Complete Edition in English*. Trans. B. Fink. New York: W.W. Norton & Co., 2006.

Lacan, J. (1960–1961). *The Seminar of Jacques Lacan, book VIII. Transference*. Trans. B. Fink. Cambridge: Polity Press, 2015.

Lacan, J. (1961–1962). *Séminaire IX. L'identification*. Unpublished seminar. Retrieved from: http://gaogoa.free.fr/SeminaireS.htm

Lacan, J. (1962–1963). *The Seminar of Jacques Lacan, book X. Anxiety*. Trans. A. R. Price. Cambridge: Polity Press, 2014.

Lacan, J. (1963). *On the Names-of-the-Father*. Trans. B. Fink. Cambridge: Polity Press, 2013.

Lacan, J. (1964). *The Seminar of Jacques Lacan, book XI. The Four Fundamental Concepts of Psychoanalysis*. Trans. A. Sheridan. New York: W.W. Norton & Co., 1998.

Lacan, J. (1964–1965). *Séminaire XII. Problèmes cruciaux pour la psychanalyse*. Unpublished seminar. Retrieved from: http://gaogoa.free.fr/SeminaireS.htm

Lacan, J. (1966). Science and truth. In Écrits, *The First Complete Edition in English*. Trans. B. Fink. New York: W.W. Norton & Co., 2006.

Lacan, J. (1967). *Petit discours aux psychiatres*. Retrieved from: http://aejcpp.free.fr/lacan/1967-11-10.htm

Lacan, J. (1968–1969). *Le Séminaire, Livre XVI. D'un Autre à l'autre*. Paris: Éditions du Seuil, 2006.

Lacan, J. (1969–1970). *The Seminar of Jacques Lacan, book XVII. The Other Side of Psychoanalysis*. Trans. R. Grigg. New York: W.W. Norton & Co., 2007.

Lacan, J. (1971). *Le Séminaire, Livre XVIII. D'un discours qui ne serait pas du semblant*. Paris: Éditions du Seuil, 2007.

Lacan, J. (1971–1972). *The Seminar of Jacques Lacan, book XIX. ...or Worse*. Trans. A.R. Price. Cambridge: Polity Press, 2018.

Lacan, J. (1971–1972a). *Séminaire XIXbis, Le savoir du psychanalyste*. Unpublished seminar. Retrieved from: http://gaogoa.free.fr/SeminaireS.htm

Lacan, J. (1972). L'étourdit. In *Autres écrits*. Paris: Éditions du Seuil, 2001.

Lacan, J. (1972–1973). *The Seminar of Jacques Lacan, book XX. On Feminine Sexuality. The Limits of Love and Knowledge. Encore*. Trans. B. Fink. New York: W.W. Norton & Co., 1999.

Lacan, J. (1974–1975). *Séminaire XXII, R.S.I.* Unpublished seminar. Retrieved from: http://gaogoa.free.fr/SeminaireS.htm

Lacan, J. (1975–1976). *The Seminar of Jacques Lacan, book XXIII. The Sinthome*. Trans. A.R. Price. Cambridge: Polity Press, 2016.

General references

APA (2013). *Diagnostic and Statistical Manual of Mental Disorders, 5th. Ed. DSM-5*. Washington, DC: American Psychiatric Association.

Aristotle (1952). Prior analytics. Trans. A.J. Jenkinson. *Great Books of the Western World. Aristotle: 1*. Edited by R.M. Hutchins. Chicago: Encyclopedia Britannica Inc.

Aristotle (1952a). Metaphysics. Trans. W.D. Ross. *Great Books of the Western World. Aristotle: 1*. Edited by R.M. Hutchins. Chicago: Encyclopedia Britannica Inc.

Bacon, F. (2000). *The New Organon*. Edited by L. Jardine and M. Silverthorne. Cambridge: Cambridge University Press, 1620.

Badiou, A. (2005). *Being and Event*. Trans. O. Feltham. London: Continuum Books, 1988.

Bettelheim, B. (1954). *Symbolic Wounds: Puberty Rites and the Envious Male*. New York: Free Press.

Brandom, R.B. (1994). *Making it Explicit: Reasoning, Representing, and Discursive Commitment*. Cambridge: Harvard University Press.

Boole, G. (2009). *An Investigation of the Laws of Thought, On which are Founded the Mathematical Theories of Logic and Probabilities*. Cambridge: Cambridge University Press, 1854.

Braunstein, N. (2017). Structures cliniques ou positions subjectives. *Analyse freudienne presse*, *24*, 39–57. Doi: 10.3917/afp.024.0039.

Castanet, H. (2017). *Quand le corps se défait. Moments dans les psychoses*. Paris: Navarin/Le champ freudien.

Castel, P.-H. (2008). *Quand est donc apparue la « névrose de contrainte »? Une conjecture historique, anthropologique et psychanalytique*. Retrieved from: http://pierrehenri.castel.free.fr/Articles/contrainte.htm

Cavell, M. (1996). *The Psychoanalytic Mind: From Freud to Philosophy, 2nd. Ed.* Cambridge: Harvard University Press, 1993.

Claude, H. Migault, P., and Lacan, J. (1931). Folies simultanées. *Annales Médico-psychologiques*, *1*, 483–490.

Claudel, P. (1945). *Three Plays: The Hostage, Crusts and The Humiliation of the Father*. Trans. J. Heard. Boston: John W. Luce Co.

Coen, J. (Director). (1996). *Fargo* [Film]. PolyGram Film Entertainment.

Coen, J., Coen, E. (Directors). (2007). *No Country for Old Men* [Film]. Miramax Films and Paramount Vantage.

Coen, J., Coen, E. (Directors). (2009). *A Serious Man* [Film]. Working Title, StudioCanal and Focus Features.

Comte, A. (2000). *The Positive Philosophy, vol. III*. Trans. H. Martineau. Ontario: Batoche Books Kitchener, 1844.

Damourette, J. and Pichon, E. (1928). Sur la signification psychologique de la négation en français. *Journal de Psychologie Normale et Pathologique*, *25*, 228–254.

De Battista, J. (2017). Lacanian concept of desire in analytic clinic of psychosis. *Frontiers in Psychology*, *8*, 563. Doi: 10.3389/fpsyg.2017.00563.

Descartes, R. (1998). *The World and Other Writings*. Trans. S. Gaukroger. Cambridge: Cambridge University Press, 1664.

Deutsch, H. (2007). Some forms of emotional disturbance and their relationship to schizophrenia. *The Psychoanalytic Quarterly*, *76*, 325–344, 1942. Doi: 10.1080/21674086.1942.11925501.

Devereux, G. (1977). *Essais d'éthnopsychiatrie générale, 3rd. Ed*. Paris: Gallimard, 1970.

Durkheim, E. (2000). *Lecciones de sociología*. Toronto: Ediciones elaleph.com, 1950.

Eidelsztein, A. (2019). *Las estructuras clínicas a partir de Lacan. Vol. I. Intervalo y holofrase, locura, psicosis, psicosomática y debilidad mental, 6th ed*. Buenos Aires: Letra-Viva, 2006.

Fink, B. (1997). *A Clinical Introduction to Lacanian Psychoanalysis: Theory and Technique*. Cambridge: Harvard University Press.

Fink, B. (2004). *Lacan to the Letter: Reading* Écrits *Closely*. Minneapolis: Minnesota University Press.

Fink, B. (2014). *Against Understanding, Vol. 2: Cases and Commentary in a Lacanian Key*. Oxford: Routledge.

Foucault, M. (1988). *Madness and Civilization: A History of Insanity in the Age of Reason*. Trans. R. Howard. New York: Vintage Books.

Fraenkel, A.A., Bar-Hillel, Y., and Levy, A. (2001). *Foundations of Set Theory, 2nd. revised ed*. Amsterdam: Elsevier, 1958.

Frege, G. (1884). *Die Grundlagen der Arithmetik: Eine logisch mathematische Untersuchung über den Begriff der Zahl*. Breslau: Verlag von Wilhelm Koebner.

Frege, G. (1960). *The Foundations of Arithmetic: A Logico-Mathematical Inquiry into the Concept of Number*. Trans. J.L. Austin. New York: Harper & Brothers, 1884.

Freud, S. (1895). Project for a scientific psychology. In *Standard Edition. Vol. I*. Trans. J. Strachey. London: Hogarth Press, 1966.

Freud, S. (1896). Letter 52. In *Standard Edition. Vol. I*. Trans. J. Strachey. London: Hogarth Press, 1966.

Freud, S. (1905). Three essays on the theory of sexuality. In *Standard Edition. Vol. VII*. Trans. J. Strachey. London: Hogarth Press, 1953.

Freud, S. (1909). Analysis of a phobia in a five-year-old boy. In *Standard Edition. Vol. X*. Trans. J. Strachey. London: Hogarth Press, 1955.

Freud, S. (1909a). Notes upon a case of obsessional neurosis. In *Standard Edition. Vol. X*. Trans. J. Strachey. London: Hogarth Press, 1955.

Freud, S. (1911). Psychoanalytic notes on an autobiographical account of a case of paranoia (dementia paranoides). In *Standard Edition. Vol. XII*. Trans. J. Strachey. London: Hogarth Press, 1958.

Freud, S. (1913). Totem and taboo. In *Standard Edition. Vol. XIII*. Trans. J. Strachey. London: Hogarth Press, 1955.

Freud, S. (1915). The unconscious. In *Standard Edition. Vol. XIV*. Trans. J. Strachey. London: Hogarth Press, 1957.

Freud, S. (1925). Negation. In *Standard Edition. Vol. XIX*. Trans. J. Strachey. London: Hogarth Press, 1961.

Freud, S. (1927). The future of an illusion. In *Standard Edition. Vol. XXI*. Trans. J. Strachey. London: Hogarth Press, 1961.

Freud, S. (1930). Civilization and its discontents. In *Standard Edition. Vol. XXI*. Trans. J. Strachey. London: Hogarth Press, 1961.

Freud, S. (1939). Moses and monotheism. In *Standard Edition. Vol. XXIII*. Trans. J. Strachey. London: Hogarth Press, 1961.

Goody, J. (2001). *The Logic of Writing and the Organization of Society*. Cambridge: Cambridge University Press, 1986.

Gómez Camarena, C. (2018). *Poème et mathème dans la clinique psychanalytique* [Doctoral thesis]. Paris: Université Sorbonne Paris Cité and Université Paris Diderot 7.

Grigg, R. (2006). Beyond the Oedipus complex. In J. Clemens and R. Grigg (eds.), *Jacques Lacan and the Other Side of Psychoanalysis: Reflections on* Seminar XVII, (pp. 50–68). Durham: Duke University Press.

Guinn, J. (2017). *The Road to Jonestown: Jim Jones and People's Temple*. London: Simon & Schuster.

Heidegger, M. (1977). The word of Nietzsche: "God is dead". In M. Heidegger, *The Question Concerning Technology and Other Essays*, (pp. 53–112). Trans. W. Lovitt. New York: Harper & Row, 1941.

Heidegger, M. (2012). *Bremen and Freiburg Lectures: Insight into That Which Is* and *Basic Principles of Thinking*. Trans. A.J. Mitchell. Bloomington: Indiana University Press, 1994.

Hornung, E. (2001). *Akhenaten and the Religion of Light*. Trans. D. Lorton. Ithaca: Cornell University Press, 1995.

Husserl, E. (1973). *Experience and Judgement: Investigations in a Genealogy of Logic*. Trans. J.S. Churchill and K. Ameriks. London: Routledge & Kegan Paul, 1948.

Hyppolite, J. (1954). Appendix I. A spoken commentary of Freud's "Verneinung". In J. Lacan, Écrits, *The First Complete Edition in English*. Trans. B. Fink. New York: W.W. Norton & Co., 2006.

Johnson, W.R. (1996). Amenhotep III and Amarna: Some new considerations. *The Journal of Egyptian Archaeology*, *82*, 65–82. Doi: 10.1177/030751339608200112.

Katan, M. (1950). Structural aspects of a case of schizophrenia. *The Psychoanalytic Study of the Child*, *5*(1), 175–211. Doi: 10.1080/00797308.1950.11822891.

King James Bible. Online. Original work published in 1611. Retrieved from: https://www.kingjamesbibleonline.org/

Lefort, R., and Lefort, R. (1988). *Les structures de la psychose. L'Enfant au loup et le Président*. Paris: Éditions du Seuil.

Lemaire, A. (1977). *Jacques Lacan*. Trans. D. Macey. London: Routledge & Kegan Paul, 1970.

Lerner, G. (1986). *The Creation of Patriarchy*. Oxford: Oxford University Press.

Lévi-Strauss, C. (1963). *Structural Anthropology*. Trans. C. Jacobson and B. Grundfest Schoepf. New York: Basic Books, 1958.

Lévi-Strauss, C. (1971). *The Elementary Structures of Kinship*. Trans. J.H. Bell, J.R. von Sturmer, and R. Needham. Boston: Beacon Press, 1967.

Lévi-Strauss, C. (1987). *Introduction to the Work of Marcel Mauss*. Trans. F. Baker. London: Routledge & Kegan Paul, 1950.

Lévi-Strauss, C. (2021). *Wild Thought*. Trans. J. Mehlman and J. Leavitt. Chicago: The University of Chicago Press, 1962.

Lipovetsky, G. (2000). *La era del vacío: Ensayos sobre el individualismo contemporáneo*. Trans. J. Vinyoli and M. Pendanx. Barcelona: Anagrama editores, 1983.

Littlewood, R. and Dein, S. (2013). Did Christianity lead to schizophrenia? Psychosis, psychology and self-reference. *Transcultural Psychiatry*, *50*(3), 397–420. Doi: 10.1177/1363461513489681.

Londoño, D.E. (2016). The emergence of psychiatric semiology during the Age of Revolution: Evolving concepts of 'normal' and 'pathological'. *History of Psychiatry*, *27*(2), 121–136. Doi: 10.1177/0957154X16629044.

Londoño, D.E. (2017). Cénesthésie et perturbations sensori-motrices comme des mécanismes générateurs de la folie: l'histoire d'un concept à l'intérieur de la psychiatrie française. *L'évolution Psychiatrique*, *82*(4), 805–816. Doi: 10.1016/j.evopsy.2017.03.001.

Londoño, D.E., Gil, L.F., and Marín, D. (2023). Psychic reality articulation in nonmainstream body modifications: A single-case study. *International Journal of Applied Psychoanalytic Studies*, *20*(1), 70–82. Doi: 10.1002/aps.1773.

Lucchelli, J.P. (2010). Lacan et la formule canonique des mythes. *Les temps modernes*, *660*(4), 116–131. Doi: 10.3917/ltm.660.0116.

Lyotard, J.-F. (1984). *The Postmodern Condition: A Report on Knowledge*. Trans. G. Bennington and B. Massumi. Manchester: Manchester University Press, 1979.

Maleval, J.-C. (2000). *La forclusion du Nom-du-Père: Le concept et sa clinique*. Paris: Éditions du Seuil.

Maleval, J.-C. (2019). *Repères pour la psychose ordinaire*. Paris: Navarin éditeur.

Mahler, M.S. and Gosliner, B.J. (1955). On symbiotic child psychosis: Genetic, dynamic and restitutive aspects. *The Psychoanalytic Study of the Child*, *10*(1), 195–212. Doi: 10.1080/00797308.1955.11822556.

Mahler, M. (1965). On early infantile psychosis: The symbiotic and autistic syndromes. *Journal of the American Academy of Child Psychiatry*, *4*(4), 554–568. Doi: 10.1016/S0002-7138(09)62158-0.

Melman, C. (2009). *La Nouvelle Économie psychique*. Toulouse: Érès.

Miller, J.-A. (1977). Suture (Elements of the Logic of the Signifier). Trans. J. Rose. *Cahiers pour l'Analyse,* 1, 1966. Kingston University. Retrieved from: http://cahiers.kingston.ac.uk/pdf/cpa1.3.miller.translation.pdf

Milner, J.-C. (2021). *A Search for Clarity: Science and Philosophy in Lacan's Oeuvre*. Trans. E. Pluth. Evanston: Northwestern University Press, 1995.

Money, J., Wainwright, G., and Hinsburger, D. (1991). *The Breathless Orgasm: A Lovemap Biography of Asphyxiophilia*. New York: Prometheus Books.

Morel, G. (2011). *Sexual Ambiguities: Sexuation and Psychosis*. Trans. L. Watson. London: Karnac books, 2000.

Nietzsche, F. (2001). *The Gay Science, With a Prelude in German Rhymes and an Appendix of Songs*. Trans. J. Nauckhoff. Cambridge: Cambridge University Press, 1882.

Nietzsche, F. (2008). *On the Genealogy of Morality*. Trans. C. Diethe. Cambridge: Cambridge University Press, 1887.

Ortigues, M.C. and Ortigues, E. (1984). Œdipe africain, 3rd. Ed. Paris: L'Harmattan, 1966.

Padel, R. (1995). *Whom Gods Destroy: Elements of Greek and Tragic Madness*. New Jersey: Princeton University Press.

Pluth, E. (2007). *Signifiers and Acts: Freedom in Lacan's Theory of the Subject*. Albany: State University of New York Press.

Porge, E. (2013). *Les noms du père chez Jacques Lacan. Ponctuations et problématiques*. Toulouse: Éditions érès, 1997.

Quétel, C. (2012). *Histoire de la folie. De l'antiquité à nos jours*. Paris: Éditions Tallandier.

Ramos, J. and Ramírez, C. (2018). Introducción. In J. Ramos Arenas and C.A. Ramírez (eds.). *Ontología social: Una disciplina de frontera*, (pp. 9–37). Bogotá: Editorial Universidad Nacional de Colombia.

Redmond, J.D. (2014). *Ordinary Psychosis and the Body: A Contemporary Lacanian Approach*. Basingstoke: Palgrave Macmillan.

Regnault, F. (1985). *Dieu est inconscient: Études lacaniennes autour de saint Thomas d'Aquin*. Paris: Navarin éditeur.

Reinhard, K. and Reinhard Lupton, J. (2003). The subject of religion: Lacan and the ten commandments. *Diacritics*, *33*(2), 71–97. Doi: 10.1353/dia.2005.0023.

Sass, L. (1992). *Madness and Modernity: Insanity in the Light of Modern Art, Literature and Thought*. New York: Basic Books.

Sass, L. (2001). Self and world in schizophrenia: Three classic approaches. *Philosophy, Psychiatry and Psychology*, *8*, 251–270. Doi: 10.1353/ppp.2002.0026.

Sauret, M.-J. (2009). *Malaise dans le capitalisme*. Toulouse: Presse Universitaire du Mirail.

Saussure, F. (2011). *Course in General Linguistics*. Trans. W. Baskin. New York: Columbia University Press, 1893.

Schreber, D.P. (2000). *Memoirs of My Nervous Illness*. Trans. I. Macalpine and R.A. Hunter. New York: New York Review Books, 1903, 1955.

Searle, J.R. (2010). *Making of the Social World: The Structure of Human Civilization*. Oxford: Oxford University Press.

Stern, D.N. (1998). *The Interpersonal World of the Infant: A View from Psychoanalysis and Developmental Psychology*. London: Karnac books, 1985.

Taylor, C. (1989). *Sources of the Self: The Making of the Modern Identity*. Cambridge: Harvard University Press.

Vanheule, S. (2019). On ordinary psychosis. In J. Mills and D.L. Downing (eds.), *Lacan on Psychosis: From Theory to Praxis*, (pp. 77–102). Oxford: Routledge.

Verhaeghe, P. (2006). Enjoyment and impossibility: Lacan's revision of the Oedipus complex. In J. Clemens and R. Grigg (eds.), *Jacques Lacan and the Other Side of Psychoanalysis: Reflections on* Seminar XVII, (pp. 29–49). Durham: Duke University Press.

Zafiropoulos, M. (2002). *Lacan y las ciencias sociales. La declinación del padre (1938–1953)*. Trans. H. Pons. Buendos Aires: Nueva Visión, 2001.

Zafiropoulos, M. (2010). *Lacan and Lévi-Strauss or the Return to Freud (1951–1957)*. Trans. J. Holland. London: Karnac books, 2003.

Index

Note: Page numbers followed by "n" refer to end notes.